A COLOUR ATLAS OF RHEUMATOLOGY

Published by Wolfe Publishing Ltd, 1974
Printed by Smeets-Weert, Holland
SBN 7234 0544 1 2nd Impression 1976

General Editor, Wolfe Medical Books
G Barry Carruthers MD (Lond)

Books in this series already published
A colour atlas of Haematological Cytology
A colour atlas of General Pathology
A colour atlas of Oro-Facial Diseases
A colour atlas of Ophthalmological Diagnosis
A colour atlas of Renal Diseases
A colour atlas of Venereology
A colour atlas of Dermatology
A colour atlas of Infectious Diseases
A colour atlas of Ear, Nose & Throat Diagnosis
A colour atlas of Rheumatology
A colour atlas of Microbiology
A colour atlas of Forensic Pathology
A colour atlas of Pediatrics
A colour atlas of Histology
A colour atlas of General Surgical Diagnosis

Further titles now in preparation
A colour atlas of Clinical Cardiology & Cardiac Pathology
A colour atlas of Tropical Medicine & Parasitology
A colour atlas of Physical Signs in General Medicine
A colour atlas of Gastro-Intestinal Endoscopy
A colour atlas of Gynecology
A colour atlas of Orthopedics
A colour atlas of the Liver
A colour atlas of Respiratory Diseases
A colour atlas of Endocrinology
A colour atlas of Cytology
A colour atlas of Bone Diseases
A colour atlas of Tumour Pathology
A colour atlas of Mycopathology
A colour atlas of Accident Surgery
A colonr atlas of Urology
A colour atlas of Staining Techniques
A colour atlas of Dentistry
A colour atlas of Surgical Repair of Jaw Deformities
A colour atlas of Periodontology
A colour atlas of Children's Dentistry

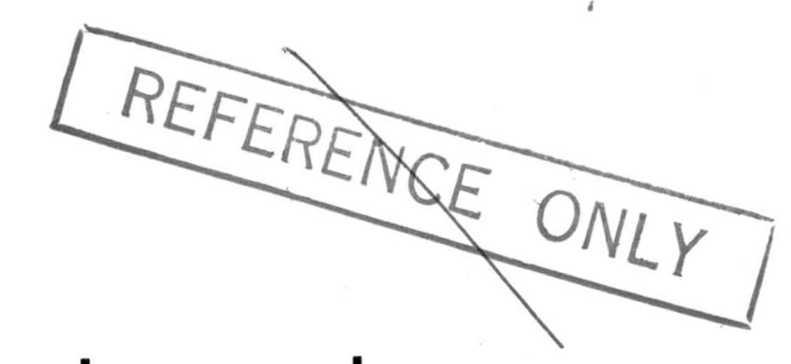

A colour atlas of Rheumatology

A. C. BOYLE

MD, FRCP
Director
Department of Rheumatology
The Middlesex Hospital
London

WOLFE MEDICAL BOOKS
10 Earlham Street London WC2

Contents

Preface

This colour atlas is not intended as a textbook, nor does it claim to be a complete record of the many manifestations of the rheumatic diseases. It simply sets out to show by clinical pictures, radiographs and histological specimens some of the more common (and a few of the less common) conditions encountered in the field of rheumatology.

Rheumatology has been one of the fast expanding fields of medicine during the past ten years, and no attempt has been made to cover the therapeutics of the various diseases described, since rapid advances in this aspect of the subject would out-date the book before publication. In addition, it was felt impossible to include the many troublesome soft tissue lesions which confront the Rheumatologist, since so few of these are amenable to illustration.

It is hoped that the illustrations will be of help to the senior medical student or the busy family doctor, neither of whom will usually have the time to delve into large textbooks for help in the diagnosis of rheumatological problems.

I am grateful to many of my colleagues at the Middlesex Hospital who have helped by providing some of the illustrations, and in particular to Professor Thackray, Dr Duncan Catterall, and Mr Peter MacFaul. Finally my thanks to members of the staff of my unit who at short notice took some of the clinical pictures as and when suitable patients attended for consultation.

A.C.B.

Introduction

Rheumatology is the study of connective tissue diseases and the medical disorders of the locomotor system.

Because pain, swelling, or stiffness of joints, or muscular pain, with or without wasting, may form part of the clinical picture of a wide spectrum of diseases, it is difficult to define its boundaries, and the Rheumatologist must be prepared for the fact that many patients suffering from diseases outside the range of his own special interest may present to him with a complaint of 'rheumatism'.

Many of the soft tissue lesions which come within the province of the Rheumatologist are of relatively small importance and are usually self-limiting, whereas affection of joints (arthritis) is a major cause of misery and crippledom in all populations.

Arthritis disables a very large number of patients, and by virtue of the fact that its course is usually protracted and progressive and that death from it is uncommon, it absorbs a substantial proportion of available medical care. In addition, as a consequence of the disability it so often causes, it may present serious social and economic problems for the patient, and on a national scale is one of the major causes of absence from industry.

Numerically, degenerative joint disease is the greater problem, but in the main is much less disabling than the forms of inflammatory arthritis. Of the latter, rheumatoid arthritis is by far the most important disease because it is so common and so often progresses to the stage when the sufferer may eventually become partially or totally dependent upon others. The list opposite lists some of the more common causes of arthritis, and in the text which follows are illustrated those which come within the particular province of the Rheumatologist.

SOME OF THE MORE COMMON CAUSES OF ARTHRITIS

Bacterial
Staphylococcus
Gonococcus
Tuberculosis
Brucellosis

Blood diseases
Leukaemia
Myelomatosis
Haemophilia
Sickle cell disease

Connective tissue diseases
Systemic lupus erythematosus
Polyarteritis nodosa
Polymyositis
Systemic sclerosis

Degenerative
Osteoarthrosis
Spondylosis

Endocrine
Acromegaly
Hyperparathyroidism
Myxoedema

Enteropathic
Ulcerative colitis
Regional ileitis
Viral hepatitis
Whipple's disease

Hypersensitivity states
Serum sickness
Drugs

Metabolic
Gout
Chondrocalcinosis
Haemochromatosis
Alkaptonuria

Neuropathic
Syphilis
Diabetes
Syringomyelia

Pulmonary
Hypertrophic pulmonary osteoarthropathy
Sarcoidosis

Unknown
Rheumatic fever
Rheumatoid arthritis
Reiter's syndrome
Psoriatic arthritis
Ankylosing spondylitis

Viral
Rubella
Glandular fever
Mumps
Measles

Rheumatoid Arthritis

In spite of intensive research, rheumatoid arthritis remains a disease of unknown origin. Although its most obvious manifestation is a sub-acute or chronic relapsing polyarthritis, it should be remembered that it is often a disease with severe disturbance of general health (malaise, anaemia, weight loss, etc.), and may be complicated by involvement of most of the body systems. Attempts to prove an infective basis for it have so far failed, nor can it be said for certain that disturbances of immune mechanisms are either a cause or an effect of the disease.

The disease is common ; figures in most populations vary between 1·6–5%. Although it may occur at any age, there is a peak for both sexes in the early forties. Women are afflicted four times more commonly than men, and in general have a poorer prognosis. Heredity appears to play only a small part in its aetiology, although familial clustering is sometimes observed.

The tendency of some clinicians to prefer the name 'rheumatoid disease' draws attention to the widespread systemic manifestations which may accompany the polyarthritis, yet to the patient these are generally unimportant in the light of progressive disablement from painful, stiffened, and deformed joints.

The essential pathological changes within the joints can conveniently be divided into four stages :

Stage I This is basically a synovitis, the synovial membrane becoming hyperaemic and oedematous with foci of infiltrating small lymphocytes. Effusion into the joint cavity will show a high cell count (5,000–60,000 per mm^3, with a predominance of polymorphonuclear leucocytes. X-rays will as yet show no destructive changes, but soft tissue swelling or osteoporosis may be seen.

Stage II The inflamed synovial tissue now proliferates and begins to grow into the joint cavity across the articular cartilage, which it gradually destroys. X-rays will now show narrowing of the joint space due to loss of articular cartilage.

Stage III The pannus of synovium having destroyed the articular cartilage by now partially fills the joint cavity, and erosions begin to appear in sub-chondral bone. X-rays will show extensive cartilage loss, erosions around the margins of the joint, and deformities may have become apparent.

Stage IV In this final stage of the disease the inflammatory process will be subsiding, and fibrous or bony ankylosis of the joint will end its functional life.

Changes similar to those found in the joints may occur in tendon sheaths and bursae. Subcutaneous nodules are often the hall mark of severe disease and characteristically contain a central area of necrotic fibrous and granulomatous material surrounded by a palisade of connective tissue cells inside an outer zone of chronic inflammatory cells. Perivascular foci of small round cells may also be seen in striated muscle and in the endoneurium and perineurium of peripheral nerves.

The most serious lesions occur in the arterial tree, sometimes presenting as a non-necrotising arteritis of the small terminal arterioles, but occasionally taking the form of a fulminating arteritis with a close resemblance to polyarteritis nodosa, and with the prospect of a fatal outcome for the patient.

Typically, rheumatoid arthritis runs a course of exacerbations and remissions, with a gradual advance of destructive changes in the joints. Nevertheless, studies suggest that up to 40% of patients have the disease in a mild form, and that it is only 10% of those affected who eventually become totally disabled.

The ultimate prognosis is notoriously unpredictable, but an insidious onset, high E.S.R. and high titre of rheumatoid factor, episcleritis or evidence of vasculitis are usually signs of serious import for the patient.

As will have been realised from the above, x-rays are usually unhelpful in the very early stages of the disease when confirmation of the diagnosis is most needed.

The E.S.R. is usually raised at the onset of the disease and is a useful monitor of activity during the years that follow. Testing for rheumatoid factor may be helpful, but it must be remembered that this test is only positive in 60% of cases, and may revert to negative when improvement occurs. A high titre at onset usually heralds a poor prognosis. A moderate to severe anaemia (the "anaemia of chronic disease"), which is normochromic and normocytic, may be found. Changes in plasma proteins are non-specific – usually a rise in the alpha 2 and gamma globulins.

The illustrations which follow are intended to show the more important manifestations of the disease.

THE JOINTS

1 Early rheumatoid arthritis of the hands Although sometimes starting as a monarthritis, this disease usually begins as a symmetrical polyarthritis, the finger joints commonly presenting the earliest manifestations of pain, swelling, and stiffness most marked in the early morning. As seen here, spindle swelling of the proximal interphalangeal joints and swelling of the 2nd and 3rd metacarpophalangeal joints are characteristic. The left wrist shows marked swelling over the ulnar styloid, and it is in this situation that the earliest erosive changes may be detected on x-ray. Flexor tendinitis in the palm of the hand is also an early clinical sign, and may be detected by palpating the flexor tendons in turn while the corresponding finger is passively flexed and extended.

2 In the early stages of the disease x-rays may be entirely normal. In sequence are : (1) soft tissue swelling around affected joints with para-articular osteoporosis ; (2) joint space narrowing due to cartilage destruction ; (3) rheumatoid erosions around joint margins.

Note well-marked cartilage loss in the left 2nd metacarpophalangeal joint, and rheumatoid erosions affecting particularly the right 2nd metacarpophalangeal joint. The carpal and radio-carpal joints of both wrists show more advanced changes, and the characteristic erosion of the ulnar styloid processes can also be seen.

This patient's disease had been present for one year when this radiograph was taken.

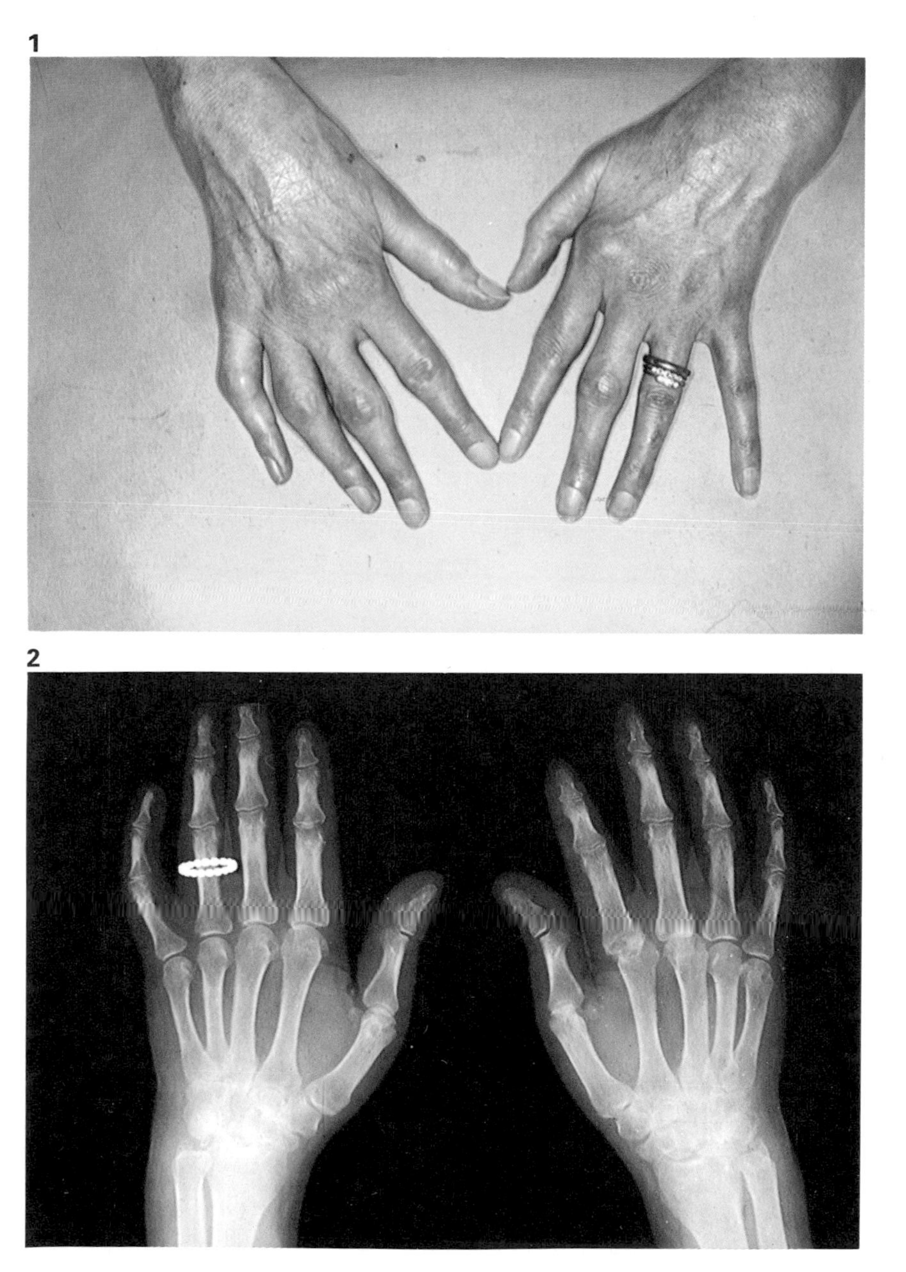
1
2

3 Severe rheumatoid arthritis of the hands Progressive and long-standing disease may result in deformity, subluxation, or ankylosis of the joints. Ulnar deviation of the fingers is typical of the later stage of the disease, and severe muscle wasting, and large tendon sheath effusions may also be seen. Note the 'swan neck' deformity of the fingers shown in this figure together with massive tendon sheath swelling over the dorsal surfaces of both wrist joints and the severe muscle wasting.

4 Late radiological signs show profound osteoporosis, an extension of destructive erosive changes with subluxation, and sometimes bony ankylosis of the joints.

5 The feet are usually affected early, presenting tenderness and swelling of the metatarsophalangeal joints. Fibular deviation of the toes may occur at a later stage.

3

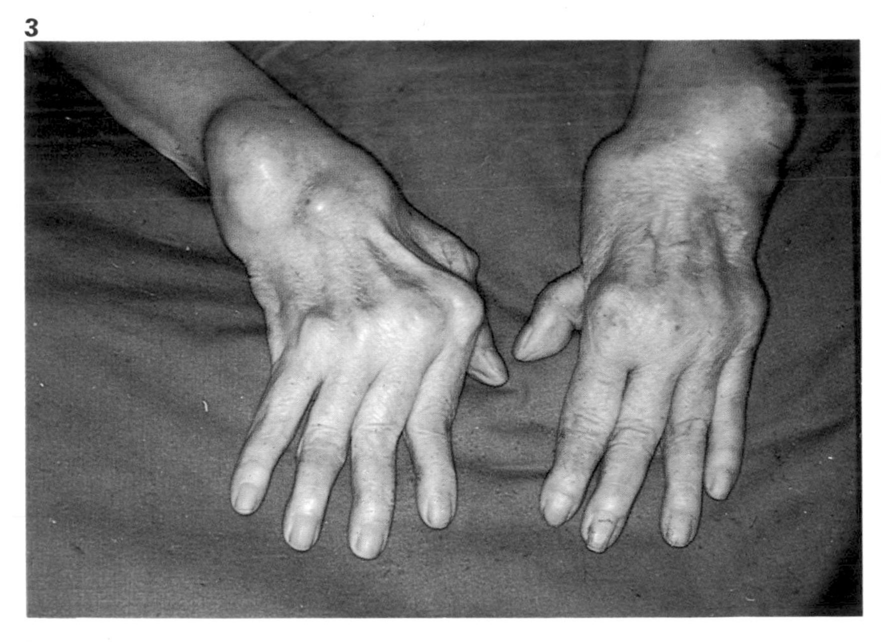

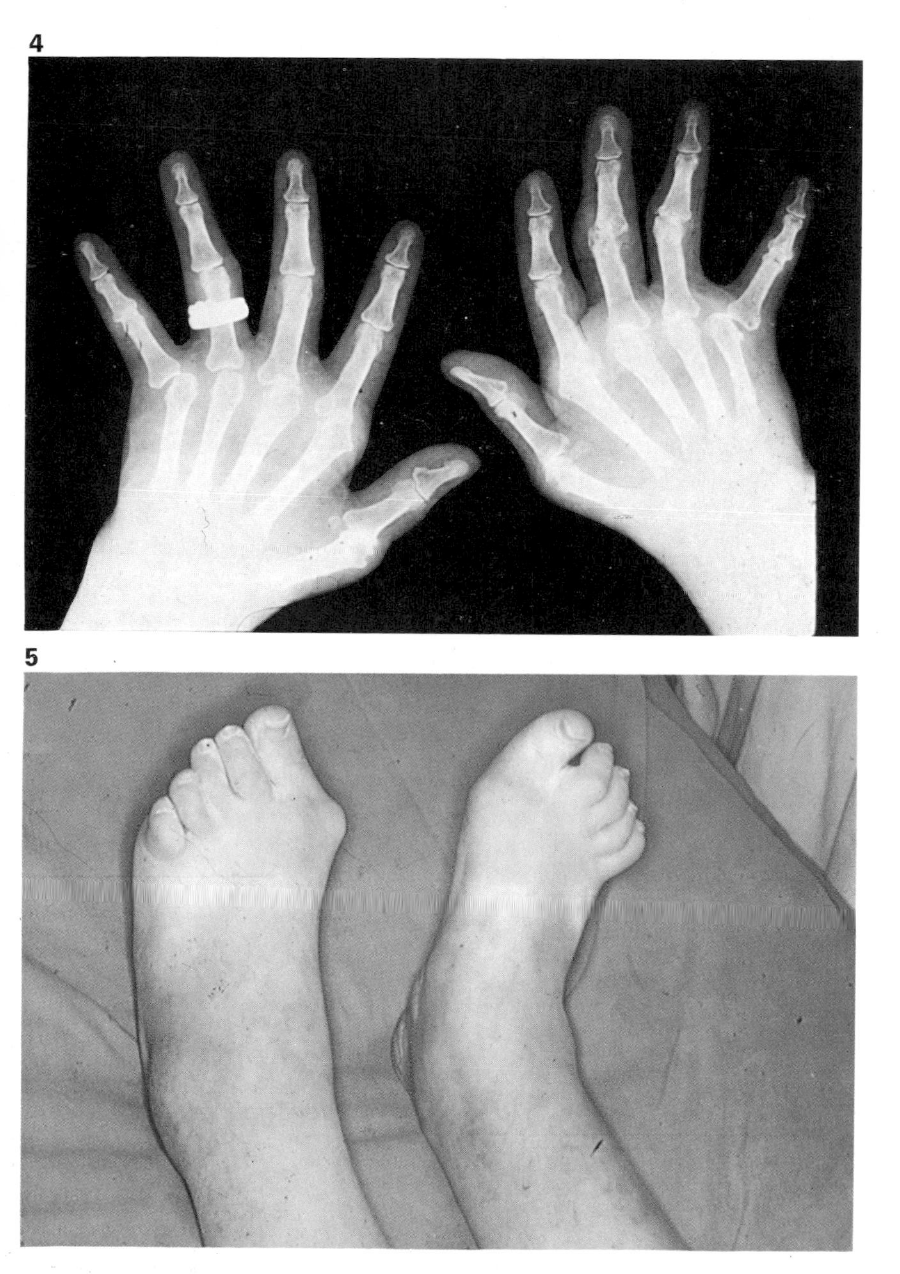
4
5

6 Cartilage loss and erosions affect the 3rd metatarsophalangeal joint. Radiological changes in the feet sometimes precede similar changes in the hand.

7 The knees are commonly involved, presenting with warmth and effusion within the joint. Flexion contracture is apt to occur early and should be carefully watched for. At a later stage lateral instability or valgus deformity may occur.

8 Advanced rheumatoid arthritis of the knee Note almost total cartilage loss and erosion of the medial tibial plateau and medial femoral condyle.

9 Rupture of the synovial membrane of the knee is not uncommon, when the effusion tracks down into the calf muscles. The patient presents with an acute painful swelling in the posterior aspect of the calf.

6

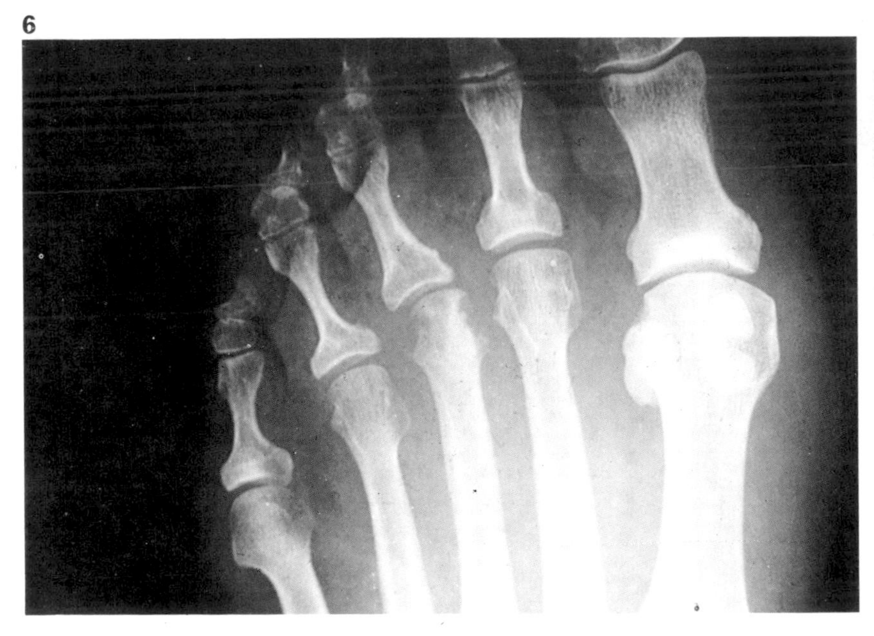

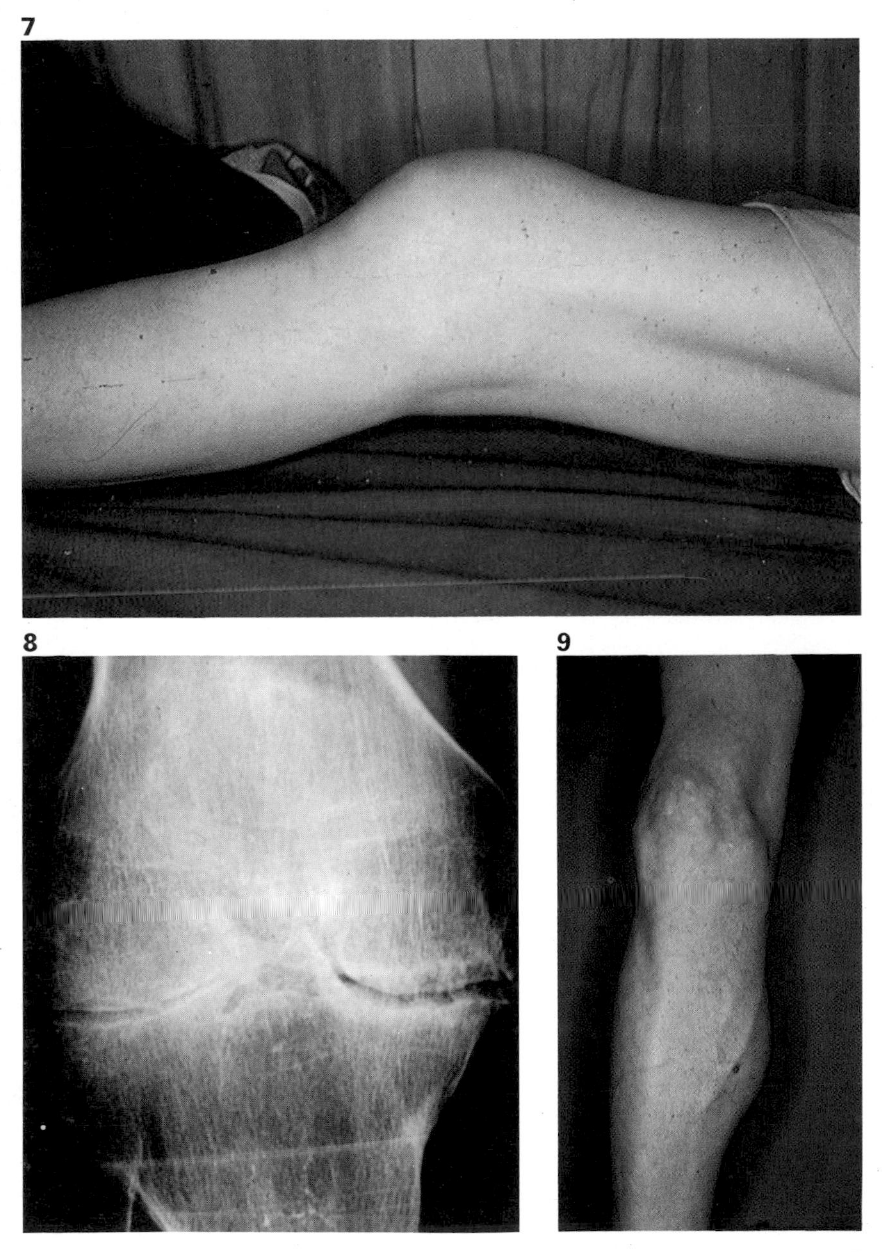

10 Early rheumatoid arthritis involving the right hip joint There is cartilage loss and erosion of the femoral head and the roof of the acetabulum. Involvement of the hip usually causes severe pain which may be resistant to medical treatment.

11 Advanced rheumatoid arthritis of the hips As with other types of inflammatory arthritis protrusio acetabuli may occur as shown in this x-ray.

12 Rheumatoid arthritis of the shoulder joint If effusion occurs, it usually presents anteriorly. Even in early involvement of the shoulder, severe restriction of movement may be present before radiological changes are seen.

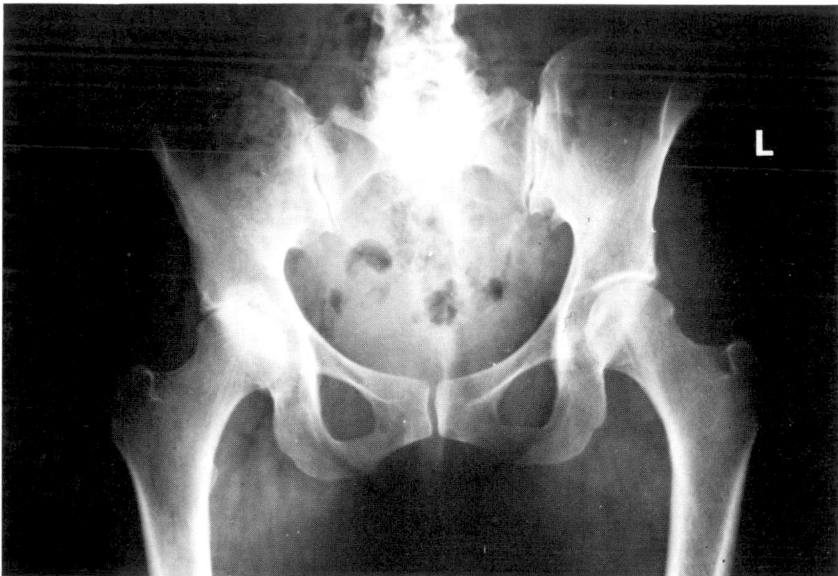

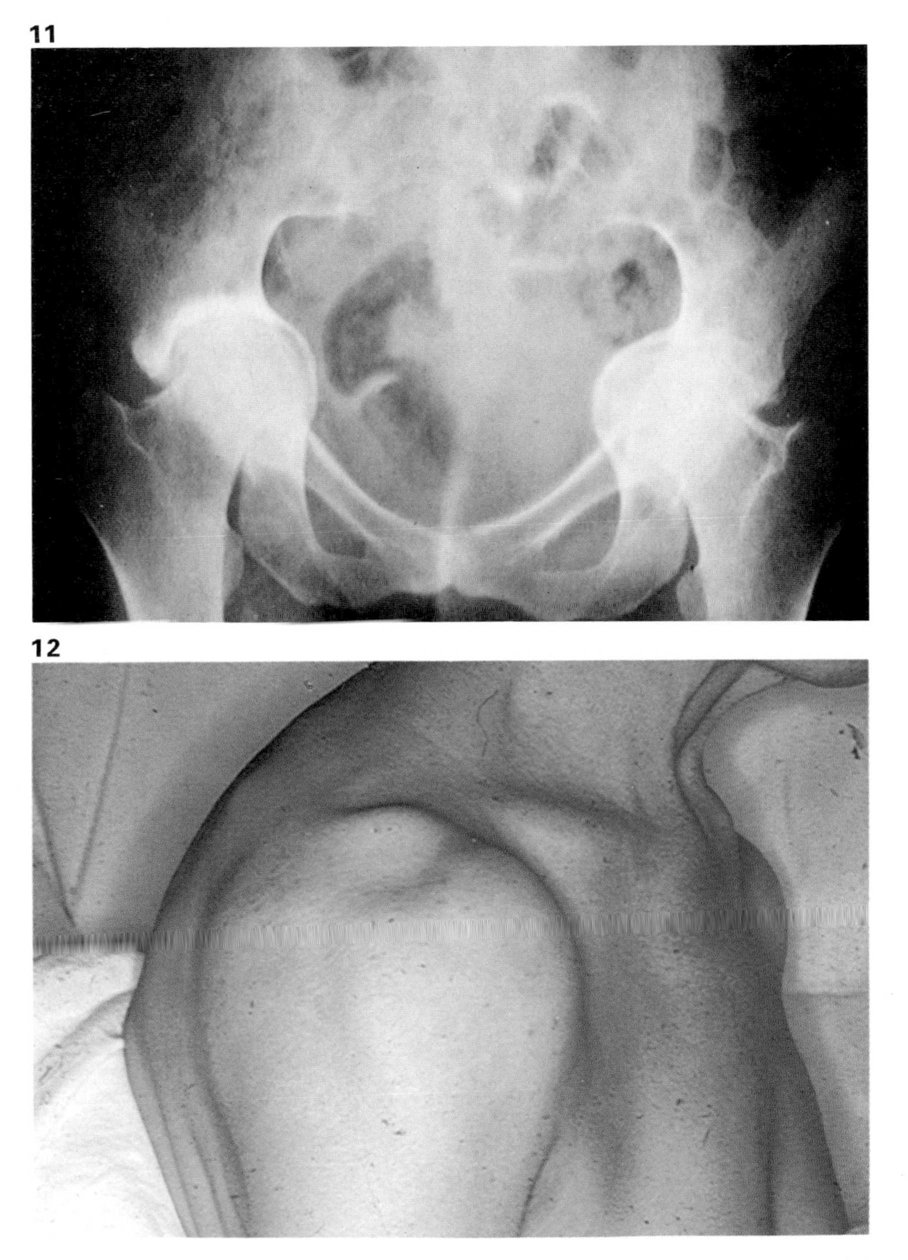
11
12

13 Advanced rheumatoid arthritis of the shoulder Note destructive changes involving the humeral head, with upward dislocation. The acromio-clavicular joint is also severely eroded.

14 Involvement of the elbow often causes considerable disability, and restriction of movement may be severe. Limitation of extension precedes loss of other movements.

15 Advanced involvement of the elbow Note almost complete destruction of cartilage and erosion of the radial head and lateral humeral epicondyle. Large rheumatoid cysts are seen more commonly in the elbow than any other joint.

13

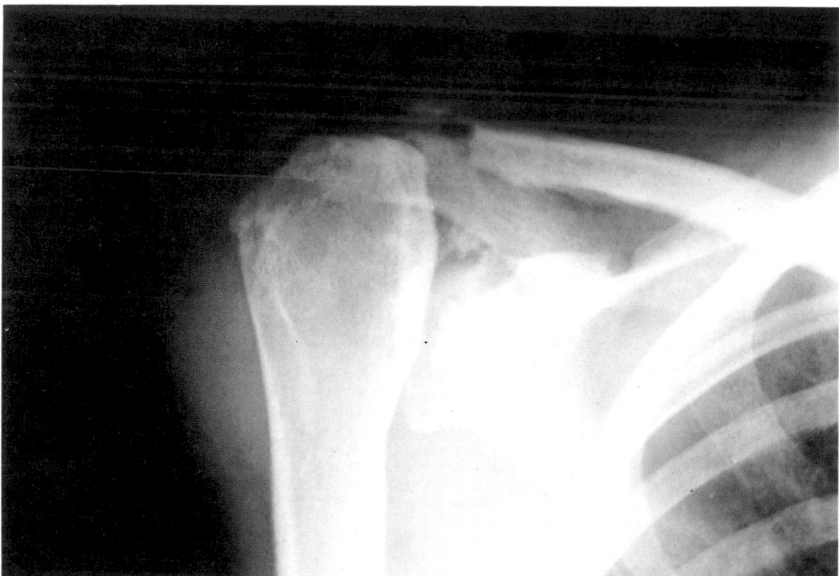

14

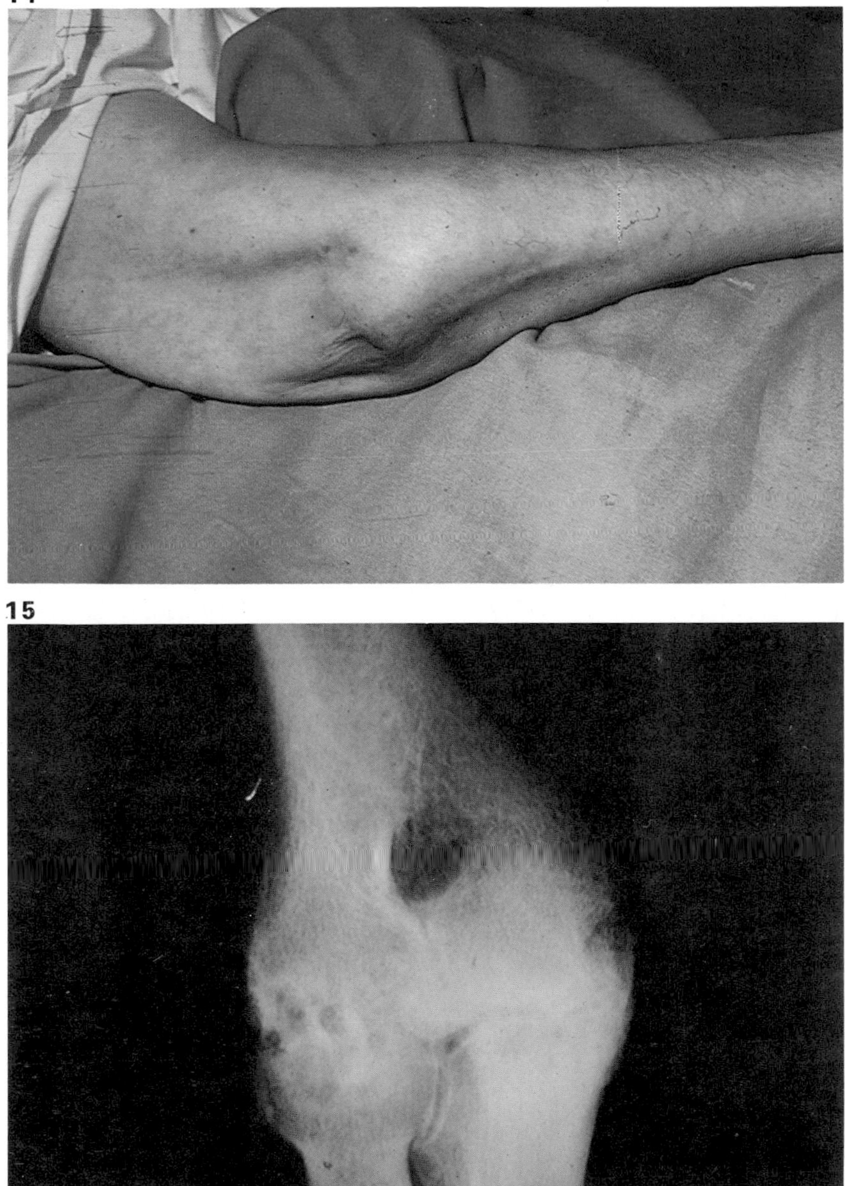

15

16 The cervical spine is the only segment of the vertebral column which may be involved in rheumatoid arthritis. X-rays taken in extension and in flexion are essential to demonstrate instability. This x-ray taken in extension shows thinning of the C.3–4 disc, with some backward subluxation of the body of C.3 on C.4. Note that the atlanto-axial joint appears normal in this view ; the distance between the anterior edge of the odontoid and the posterior edge of the arch of the atlas not exceeding the normal 3mm.

17 The same patient in flexion position Gross instability of the atlanto-axial joint is now seen, as the distance between the anterior border of the odontoid and the posterior arch of the atlas has increased to 8mm. Instability of any segment of the cervical spine may lead to cord compression with consequent myelopathy, usually a spastic tetraparesis. Multi-radicular lower motor neurone signs may also be present in the arms.

18 Advanced rheumatoid arthritis of the cervical spine with partial destruction of discs between C.4–5 and C.5–6. Note the absence of osteophytes, and erosion of the upper border of C.5, features which distinguish this condition from cervical spondylosis. Note also that this patient has had an occipito-cervical fusion for atlanto-axial instability.

19 Autopsy specimen of a patient who died from the consequences of cervical cord compression due to rheumatoid arthritis. Note major compression of the cervical cord at C.4–5 level.

Quite severe atlanto-axial subluxations may occur in the absence of myselopathy, whereas minor degrees of subluxation at lower levels may compress the cord. This is because the cervical canal widens appreciably above the body of C.2, as can be well seen in this illustration.

16

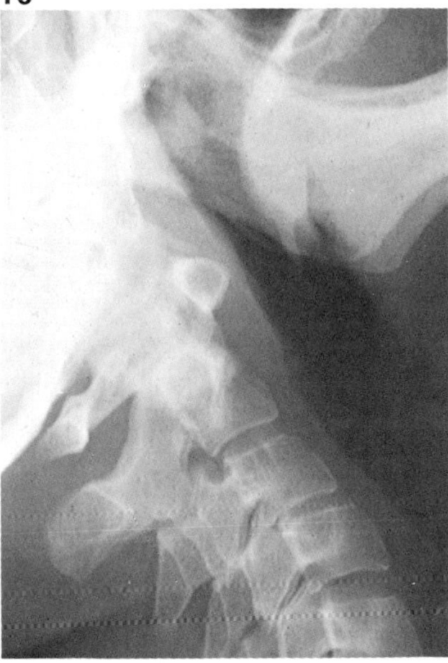

17

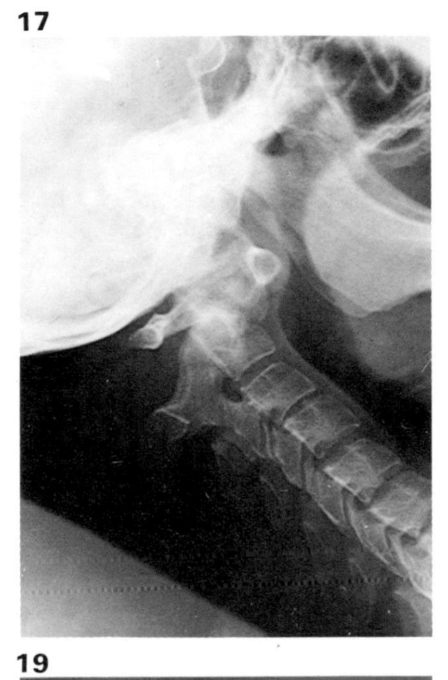

18

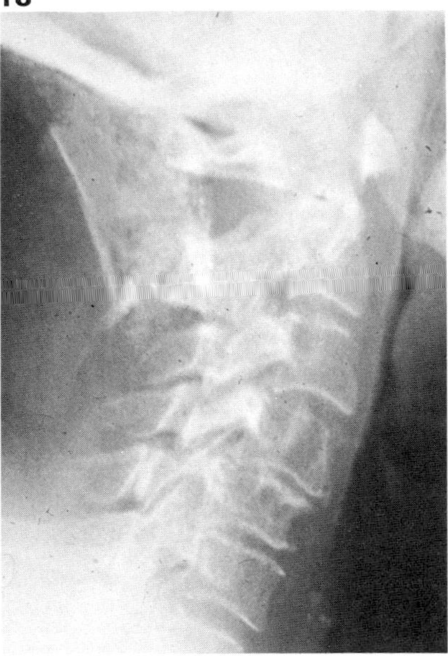

19

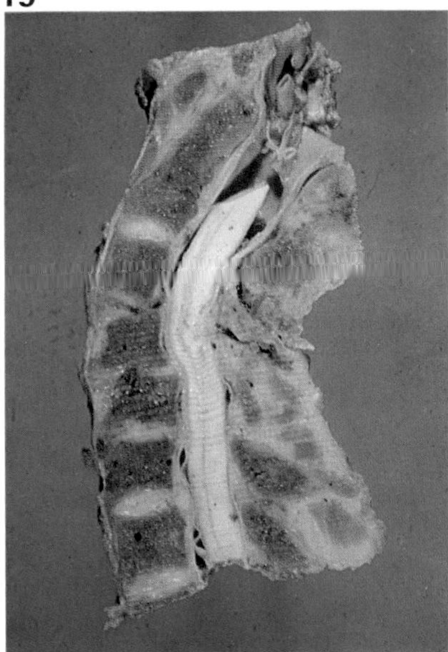

20 Pyarthrosis of the shoulder The joint affected by rheumatoid arthritis is unduly susceptible to infection – usually by the staphylococcus. An unwary clinician may accept a sudden exacerbation of pain and swelling to be due to an increase of rheumatoid activity within the joint if this is not borne in mind. Early diagnosis of a pyarthrosis is essential, since destructive changes occur with alarming rapidity, and in addition the condition may be life threatening. Any rheumatoid joint presenting with severe inflammatory signs and an undue degree of pain should be suspected of being infected, and aspirated fluid sent for bacteriological examination. Accompanying systemic signs, such as fever and leucocytosis, should be looked for.

This illustration shows such a condition, and pus has already tracked down the upper arm.

21 Severe destructive changes in a pyarthrosis Three weeks after the diagnosis of pyarthrosis was made almost total destruction of the humeral head and glenoid has occurred.

22 Pyarthrosis of the elbow joint complicating rheumatoid arthritis. Again severe destructive changes are shown.

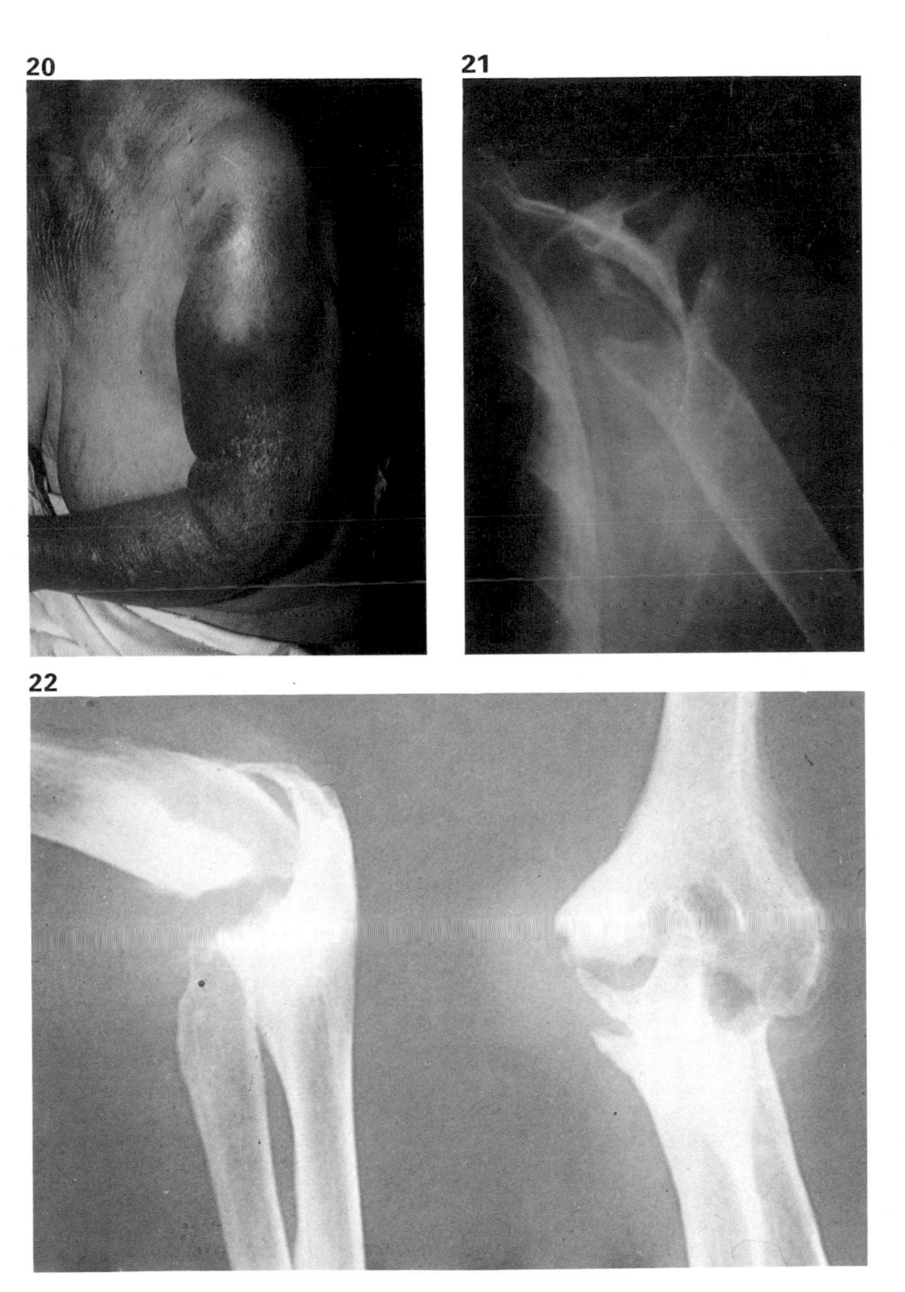
20
21
22

TENDONS AND MUSCLES

23 Effusion in the sheath overlying the lower end of the ulna Tendons and their sheaths may be involved by effusion or nodule formation. Tendon sheath swelling due to tenosynovitis is common.

24 Nodule formation in the tendon of extensor digitorum longus. Nodules in finger flexor tendons are more usual and may cause triggering of the fingers, especially in the early morning.

25 Rupture of the extensor tendon of the 5th finger Attrition rupture of tendons (usually extensor tendons) may occur suddenly, and be due to quite minor strain. Two causes are apparent: (1) softening of the tendon due to inflammatory tendinitis; (2) attrition of the tendon due to subluxation at the wrist joint, the tendon riding over roughened bone surfaces.

23

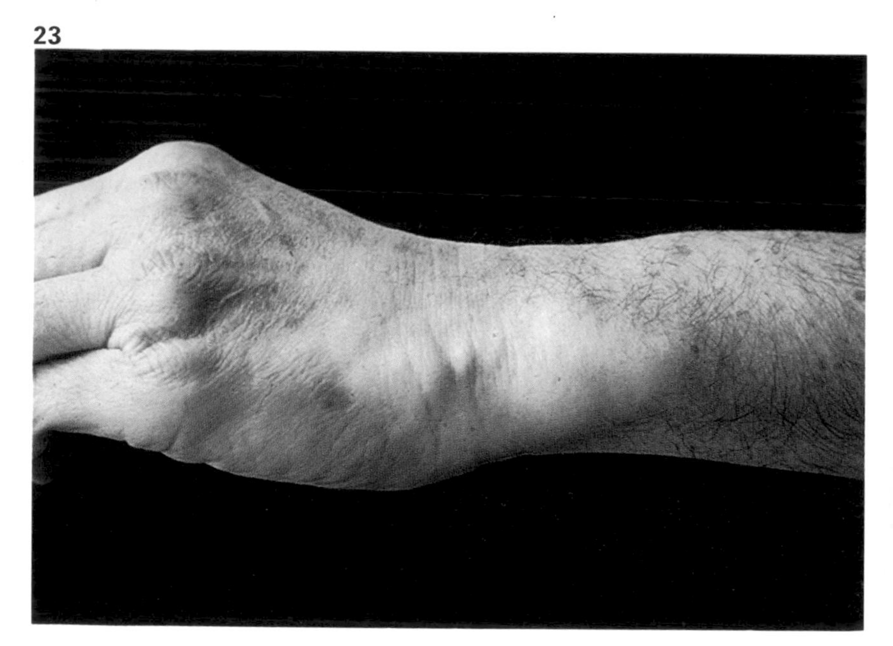

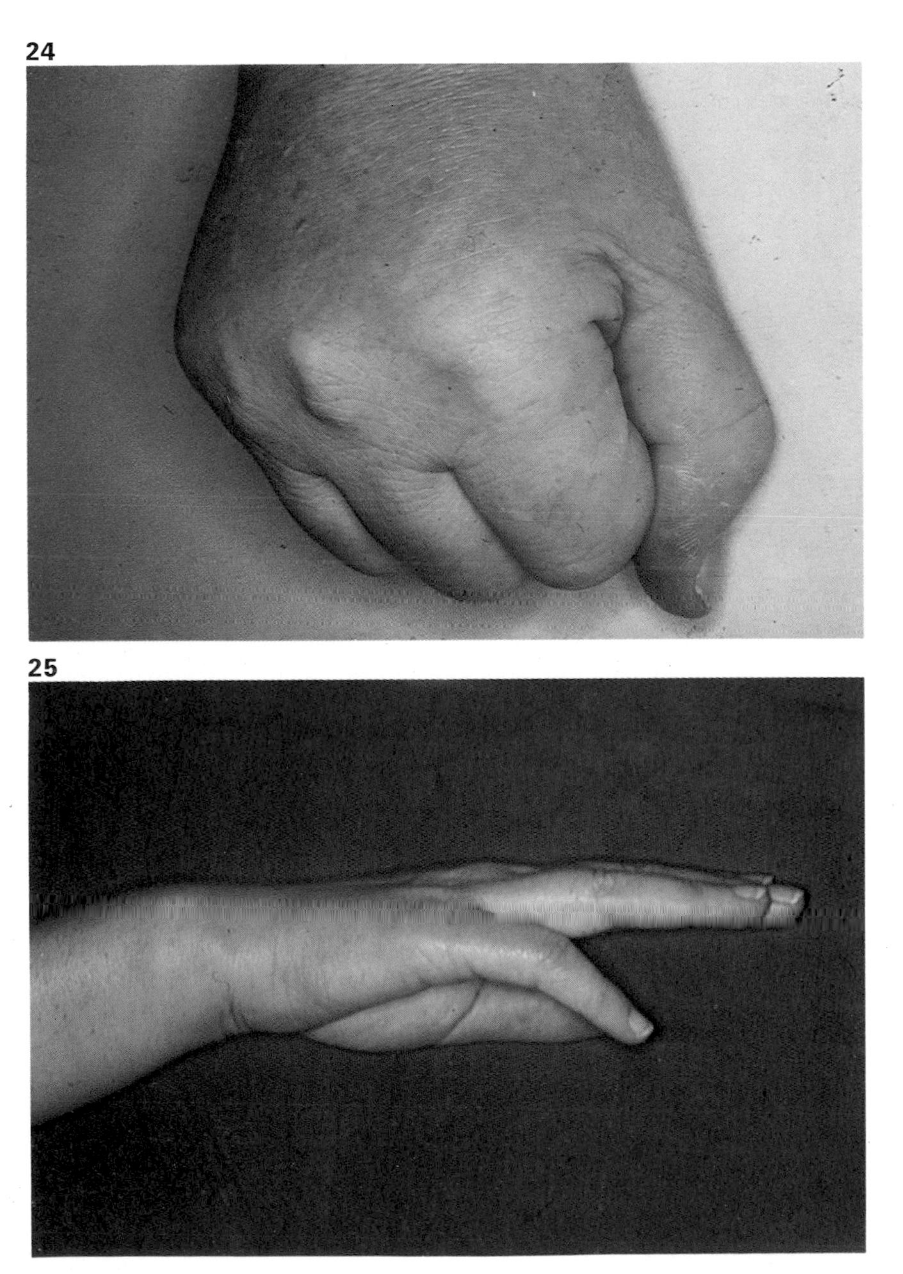

26 Rupture of two extensor tendons The widely separated ends of the two ruptured tendons are seen in the lower half of the illustration, indicating the difficulty which may be experienced in obtaining apposition at operation. The upper tendons are intact, and the probe points to a roughened spicule of bone held to be partially responsible for the attrition of the ruptured tendons. Surgical aid should be sought early, since wide separation of the tendons may make repair impossible.

27 A proximal myopathy may occur as an integral part of rheumatoid arthritis, most commonly affecting the shoulder girdle. Diagnosis may be difficult since the muscles may already be severely wasted secondary to involvement of the shoulder joints themselves. In addition weakness, giving rise to inability to raise the arms, may be wrongly interpreted as restriction due to pain.

Treatment by steroids, particularly Triamcinolone, may cause a similar condition, and distinguishing between the two causes may present a diagnostic problem.

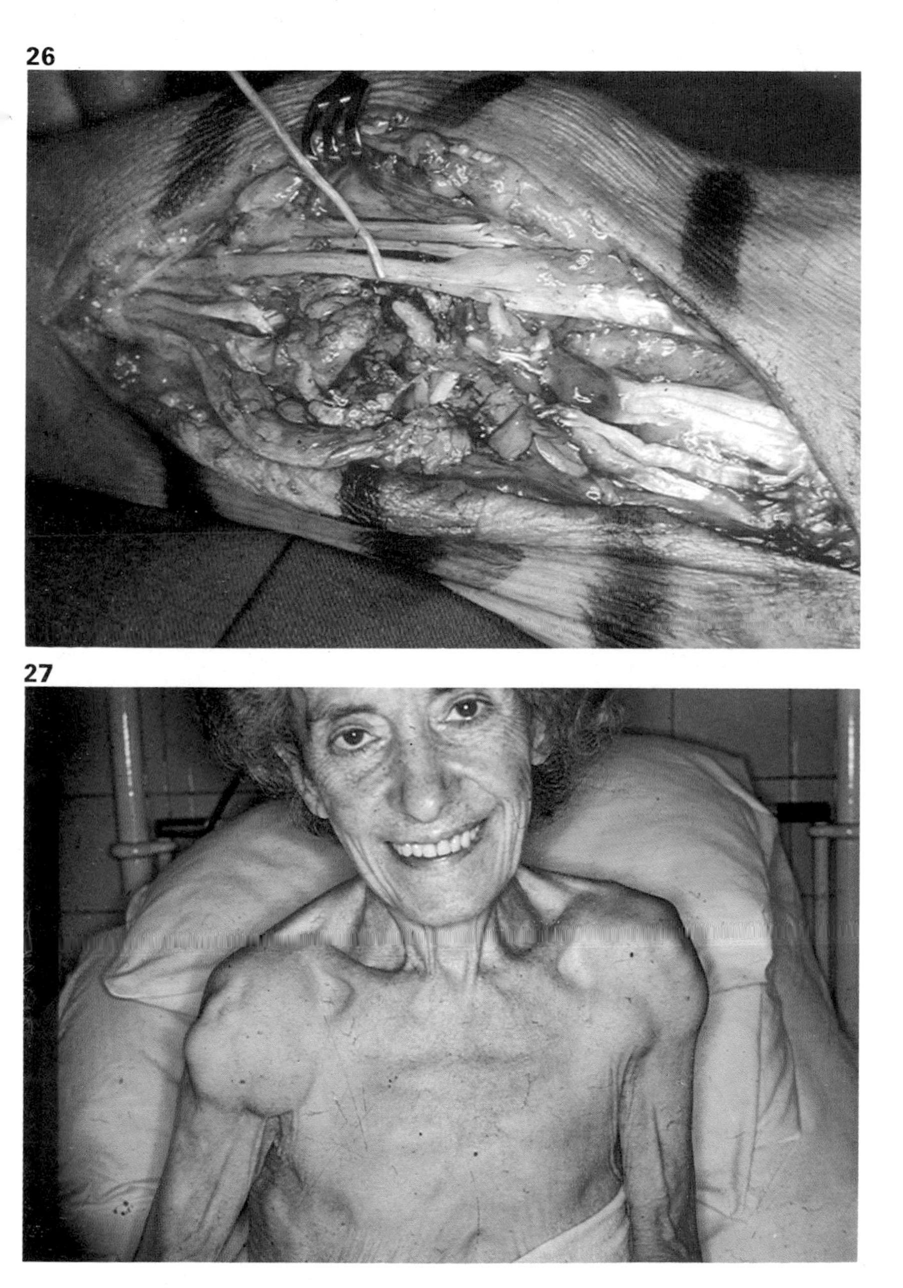
26
27

THE SKIN

28 Skin nodules occur in about 25% of patients with rheumatoid arthritis. They usually are associated with severe disease and high titre of rheumatoid factor, and generally indicate a poor prognosis. The elbow is their most common site, and necrosis of the nodule may occur.

29 The Achilles tendon is another common site of nodule formation.

30 Ulcers on the lower leg are common and probably have a multiple aetiology. The skin in rheumatoid arthritis is thin and atrophic and easily damaged, while the peripheral circulation is poor due to stasis. Some of these ulcers undoubtedly have an arteritic basis (see section on cardio-vascular complications).

31 Drug eruptions Although a rash is not a feature of adult rheumatoid arthritis (see Still's disease p. 48), skin eruptions are not uncommon as a result of drug treatment – notably by gold (of which this is an example), D-Penicillamine and Alclofenac among others.

28

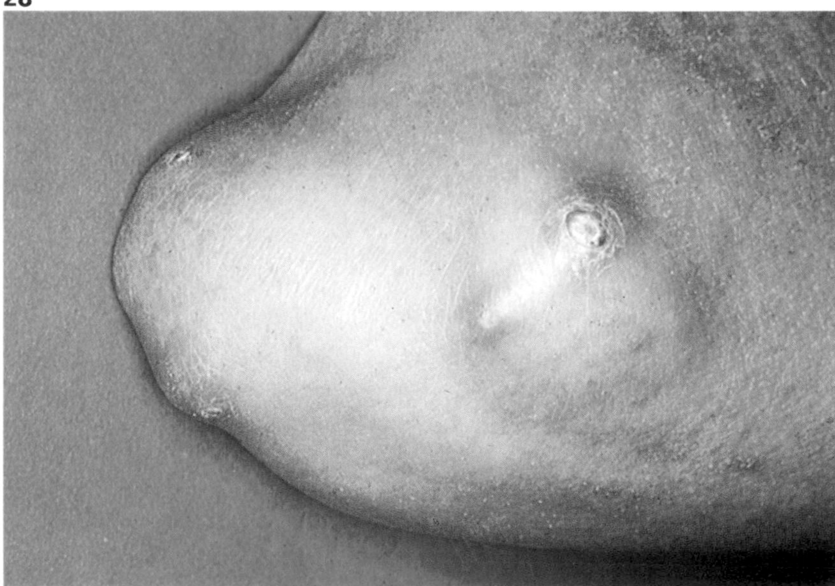

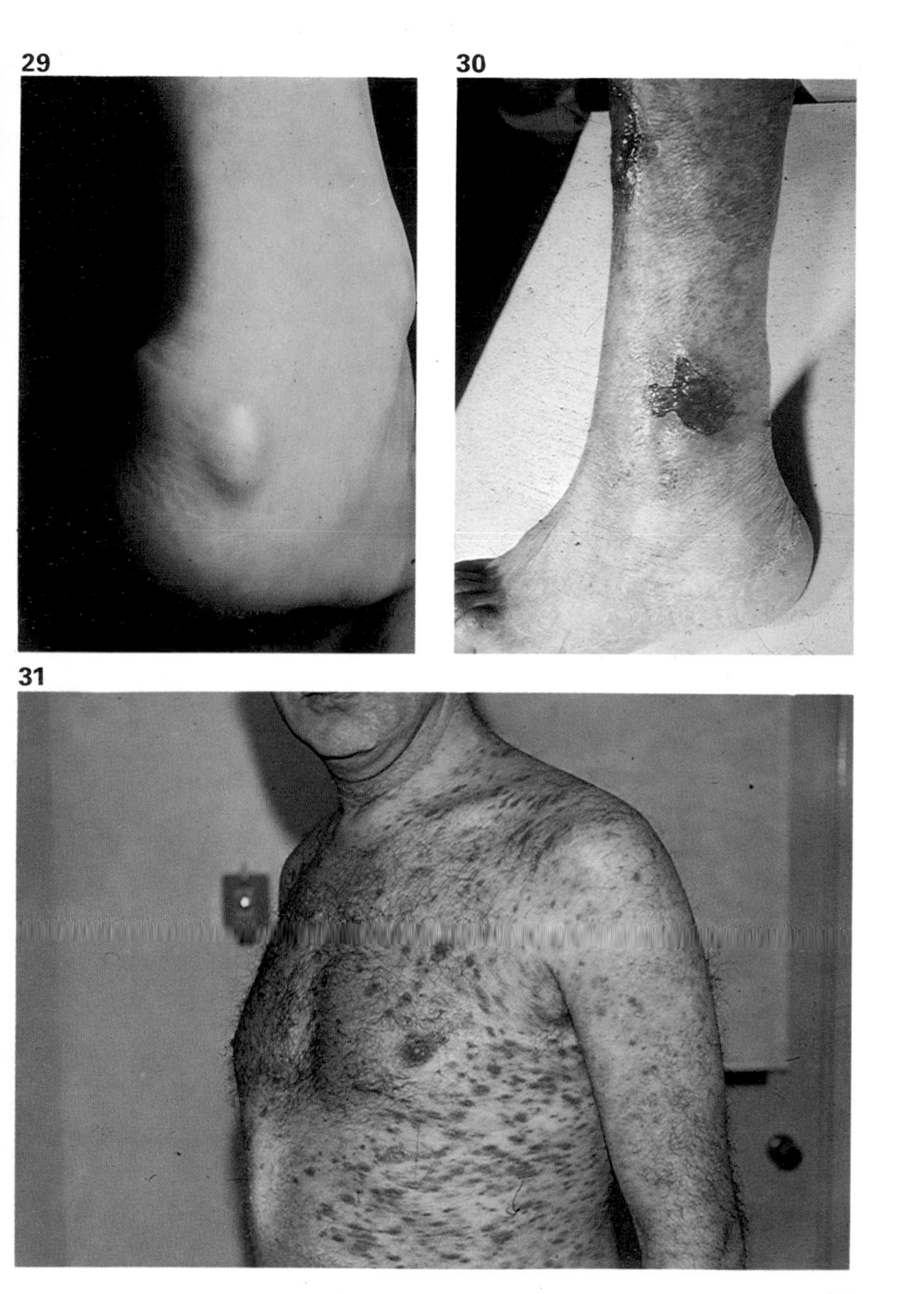
29
30
31

THE EYES

32 Rheumatoid scleritis is the most common ocular complication of rheumatoid arthritis, and generally indicates a poor prognosis. It is often associated with skin nodules, and a high titre of rheumatoid factor. The incidence of iritis in rheumatoid arthritis is no greater than that found in the general population.

33 Nodular scleritis is a more advanced stage of the previous case.

34 Scleromalacia perforans At a later stage nodules which have formed in the sclera may break down giving rise to ulceration. As with scleritis, this is usually associated with severe disease and skin nodules, and carries a poor prognosis.

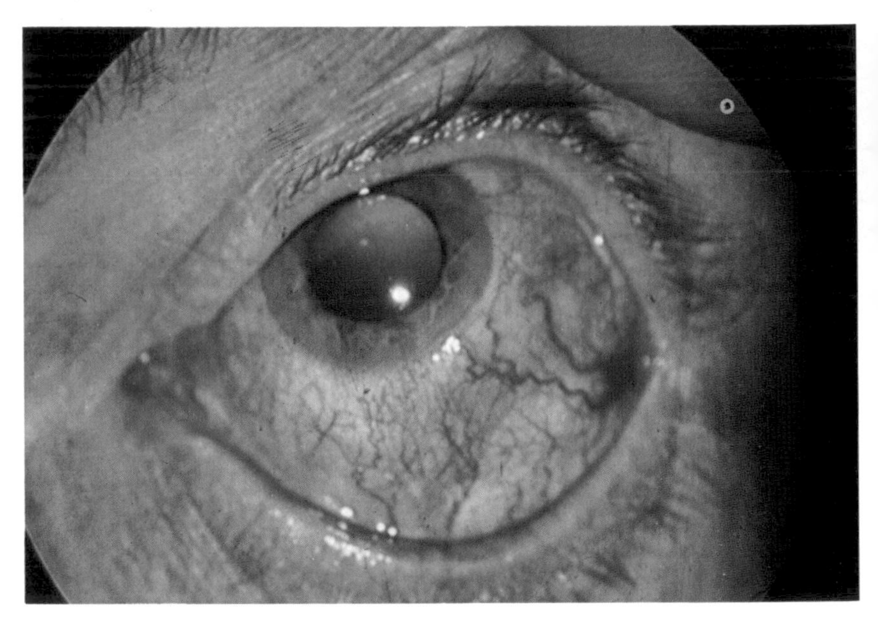

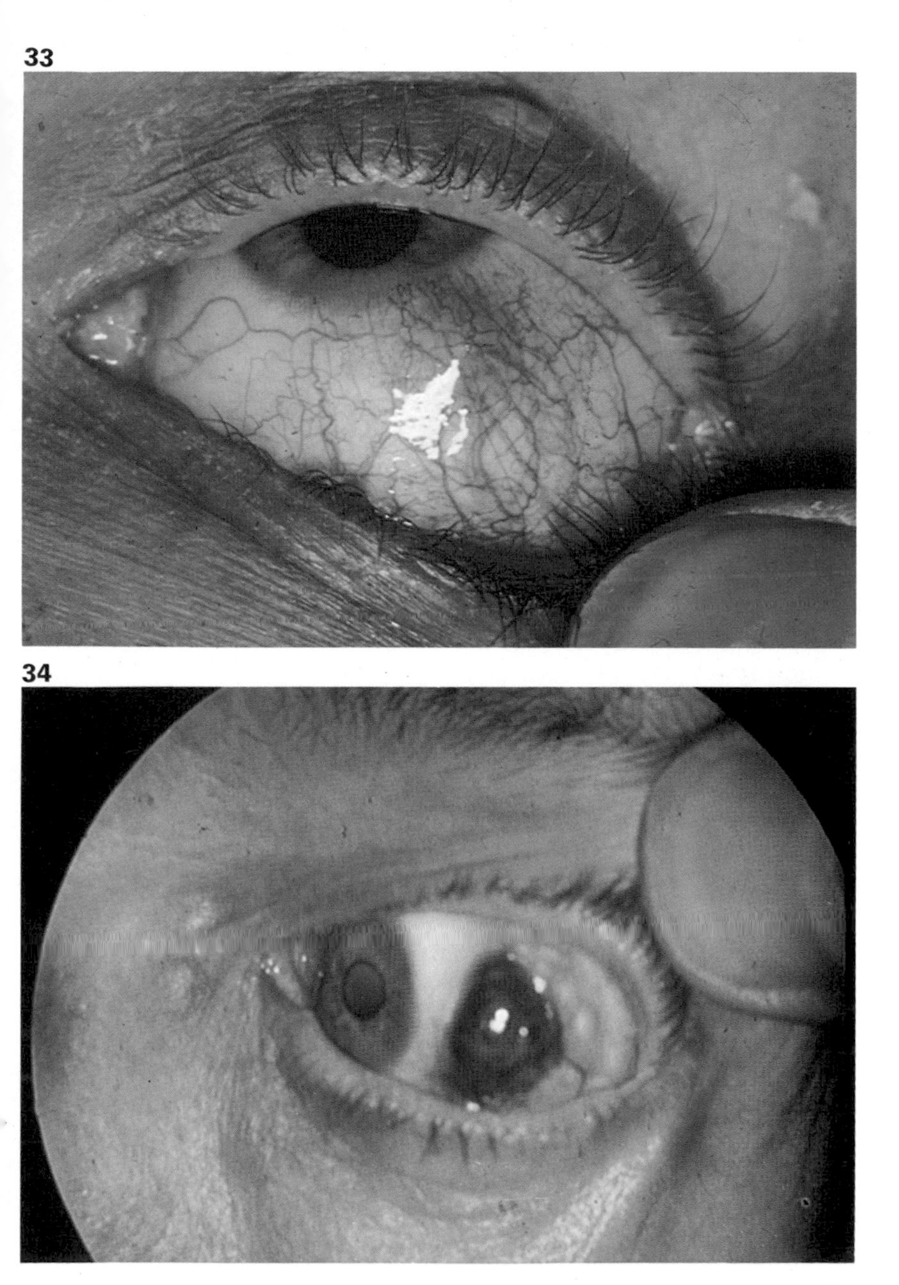
33
34

35 Sjogren's syndrome (kerato-conjunctivitis sicca) may occur in other connective tissue disorders, especially progressive systemic sclerosis. Dryness of the eyes and mouth is characteristic, and lack of bronchial secretion and atrophic gastritis may occur. Deficient lachrymal secretion may be tested for by Schirmer's test, but staining with rose bengal is more reliable. Tiny superficial ulcers take up the stain as shown here.

36 Posterior subscapular cataracts may occur, particularly after prolonged steroid therapy. Steroids may also precipitate the onset of glaucoma.

37 Chloroquine retinopathy Note the typical 'bull's eye' formation, with atrophy of retinal cells. This serious eye complaint may be induced by prolonged treatment with anti-malarial drugs.

35

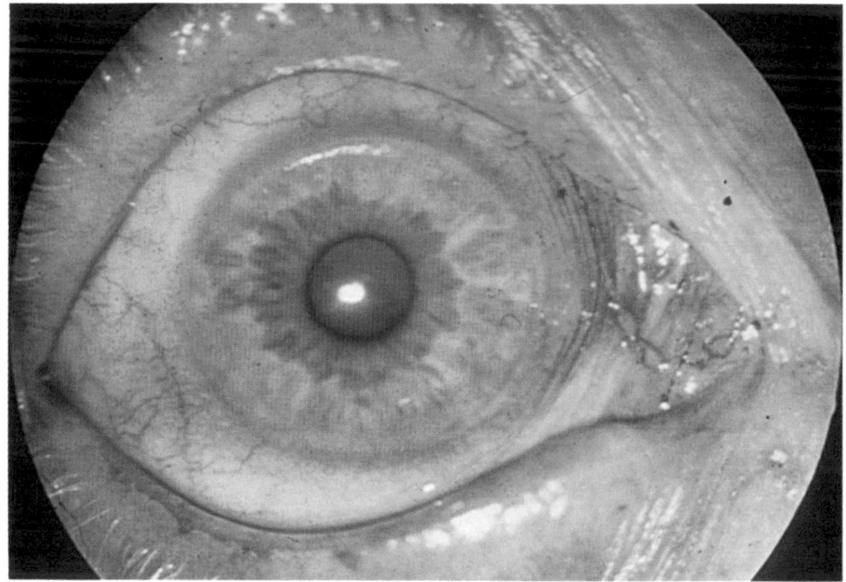

36

37

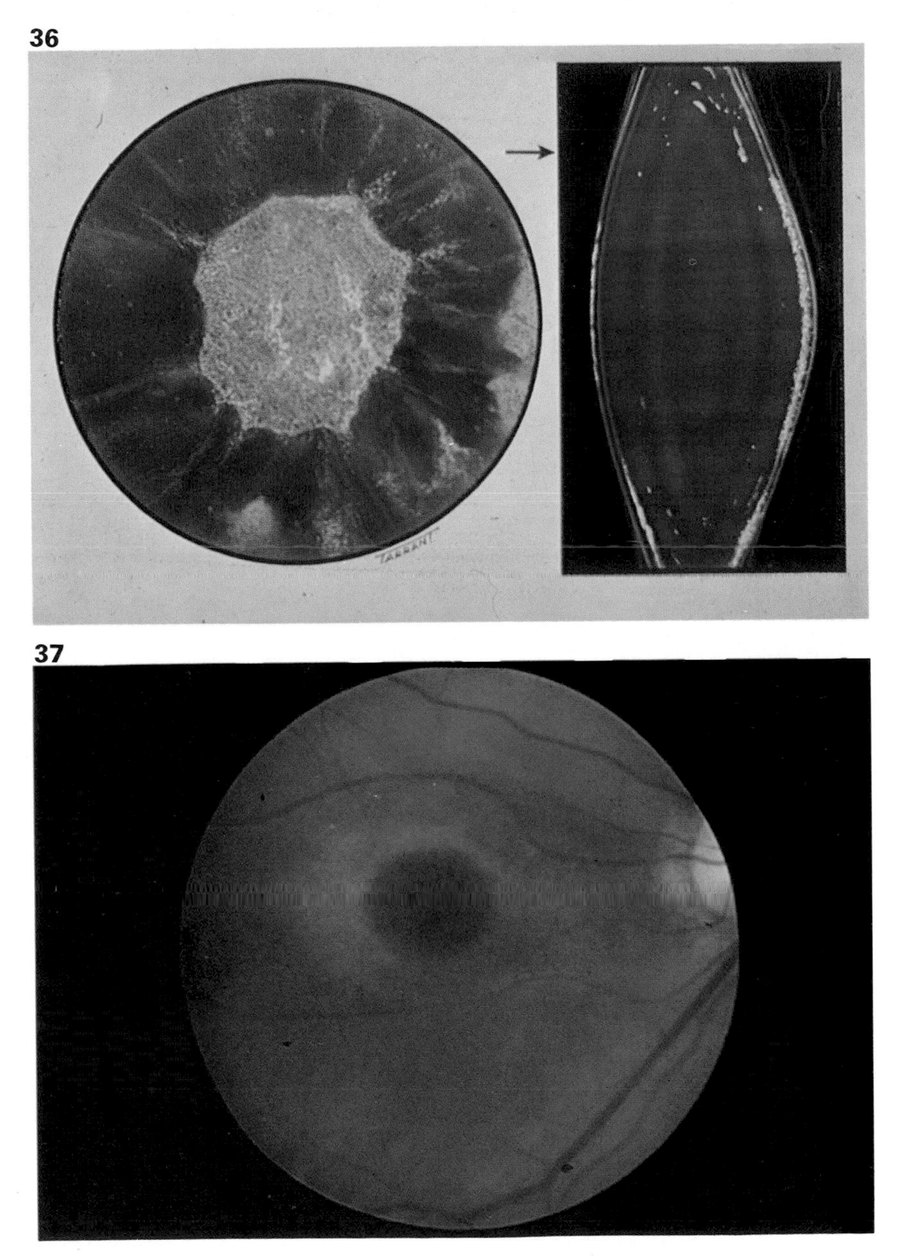

THE LUNGS

38 Solitary lung nodule in the 4th right interspace. Rheumatoid nodules may be present in the lung parenchyma or in the pleura. They may be single or multiple. Differential diagnosis from other round shadows in the lung (e.g. carcinoma) may be difficult.

39 Tomogram of the previous x-ray Note that cavitation has occurred in the central part of the nodule.

40 Rheumatoid pleural effusions may be unilateral or bilateral, and typically occur in the middle aged male. Before accepting this as a manifestation of rheumatoid arthritis, other causes of effusions must be excluded. These effusions (unless large or bilateral or both) are often symptomless, and many of them resolve spontaneously. Diagnosis may be aided by the fact that a positive test for rheumatoid factor may be found in the fluid aspirated for examination.

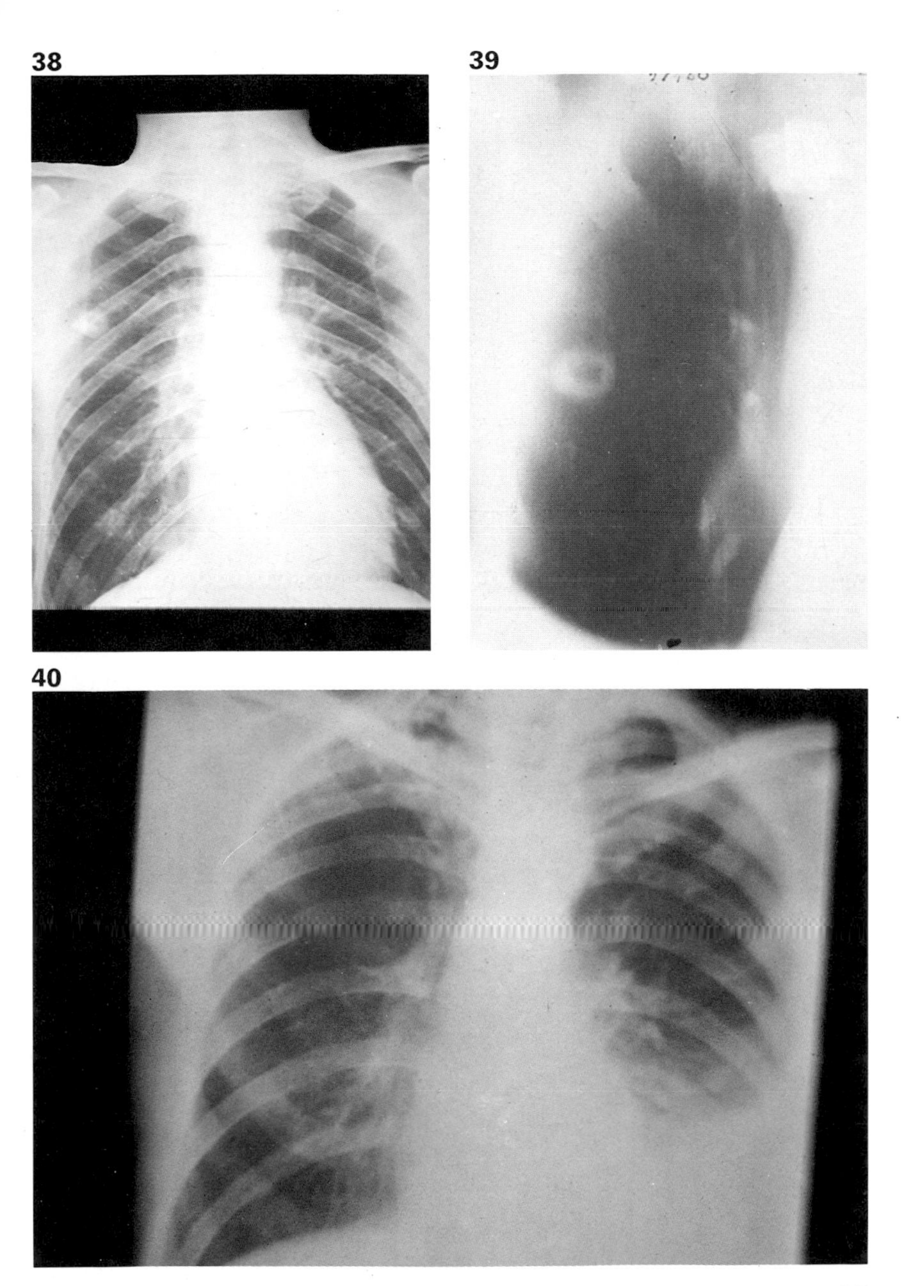
38
39
40

41 The rheumatoid lung This is a fibrosing alveolitis, at first confined to the basal areas, but may eventually involve the whole lung field. Fibrosing alveolitis not uncommonly occurs without other manifestations of rheumatoid arthritis, but many such patients show a positive test for rheumatoid factor. In some, true rheumatoid arthritis may eventually develop after the lapse of months or even years.

42 Clubbing of the fingers may be associated with the rheumatoid lung, in addition to the stigmata of rheumatoid arthritis.

43 Caplan's syndrome The association of pneumoconiosis and rheumatoid arthritis may give this picture of multiple, well-defined hard round shadows scattered throughout both lung fields.

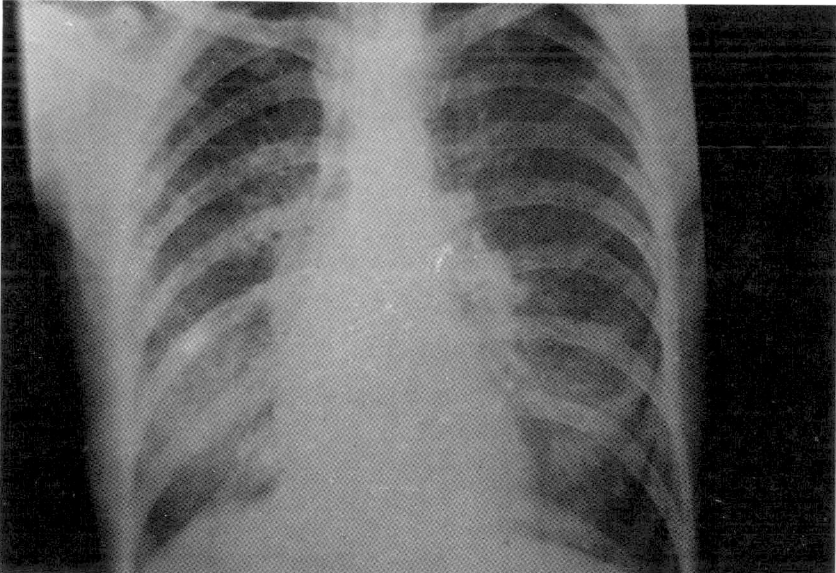

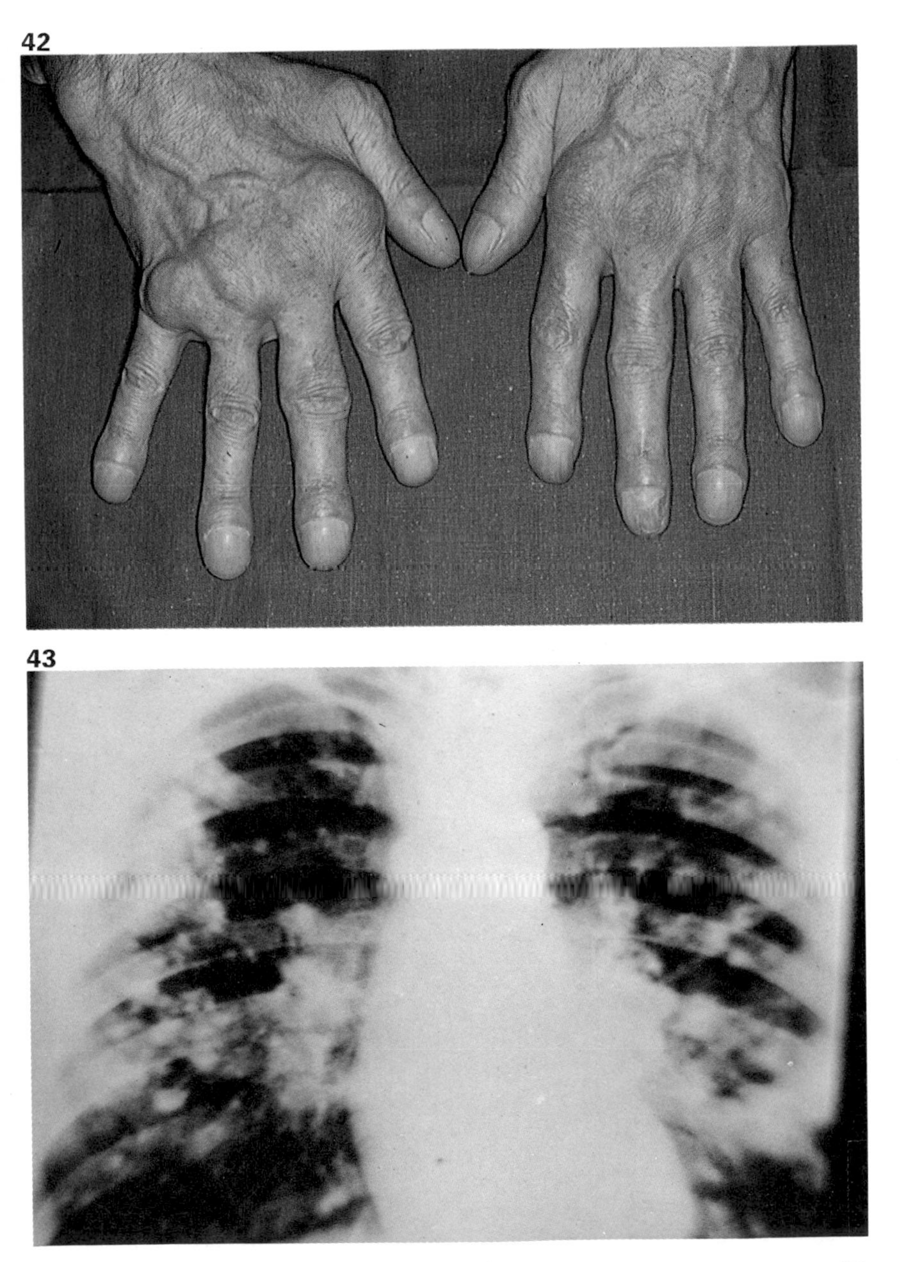
42

43

THE CARDIO-VASCULAR SYSTEM

44 Nail fold lesions are an expression of digital arteritis, and often indicate an ensuing generalized rheumatoid vasculitis. The lesion on the ulnar side of the middle finger is typical. Minor lesions are also seen on the nail bed of the index finger and little finger.

45 More advanced arteritic lesions The nail folds and both 3rd metacarpophalangeal joints are involved.

46 Advanced peripheral arterial lesions Gangrene of the digits is shown on the 4th toe, with threatened gangrene of the 3rd toe.

This degree of peripheral arteritis often heralds a fatal outcome for the patient since it is likely that the condition is widespread, involving the arterial system of all organs of the body. In such patients there is a significant mortality from ischaemic heart disease, while in others multiple gut perforation may occur due to arteritis and thrombosis of the vessels supplying the intestines. Neurological complications may include cerebro-vascular accidents or peripheral neuropathy (see **54** and **55**).

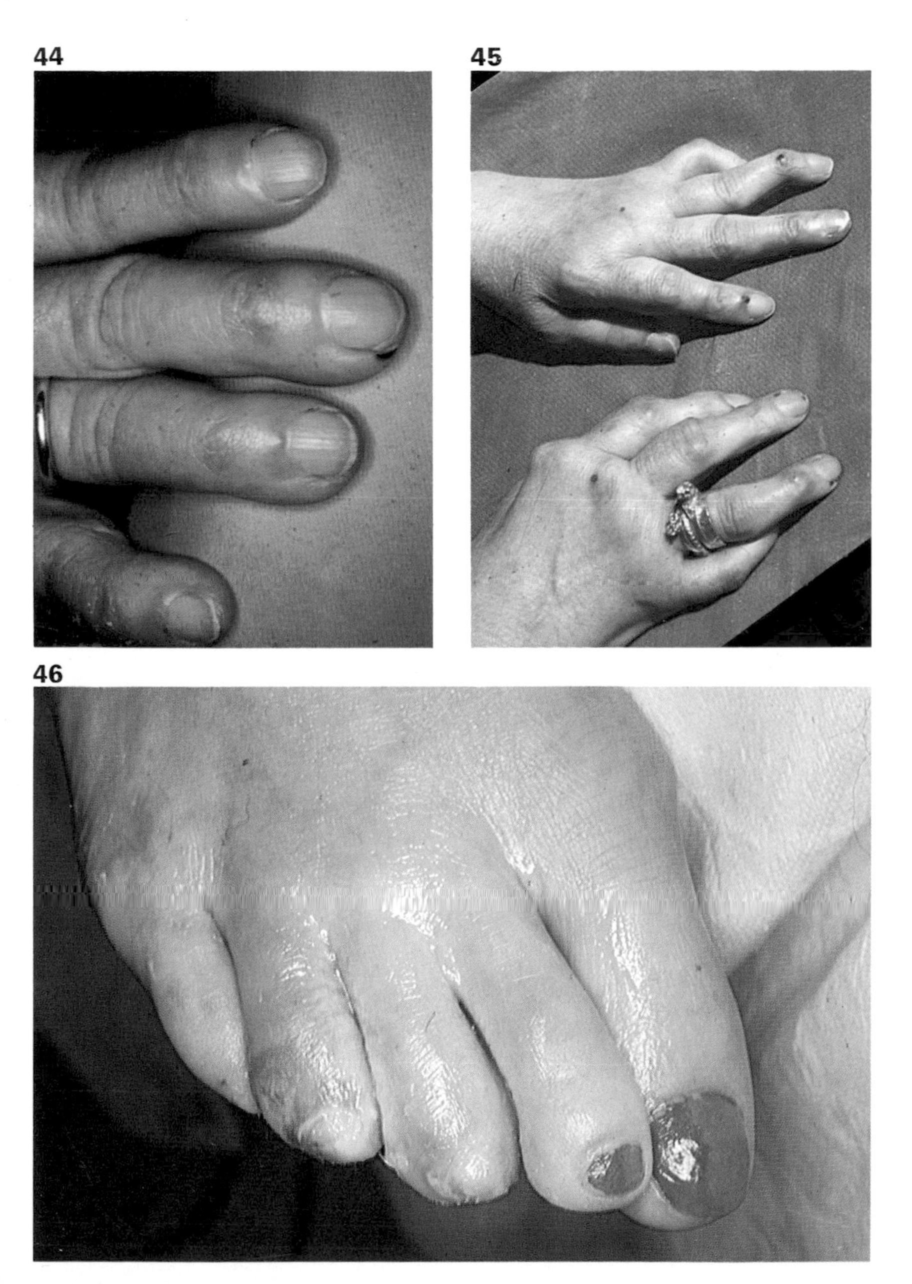
44
45
46

47 Dry gangrene of the 5th toe, due to rheumatoid vasculitis. The patient died following multiple gut perforations and a coronary thrombosis, both due to widespread vasculitis.

48 Histological presentation of vasculitis An inflammation of the intima of the small and medium sized vessels with round cell infiltration may proceed to thrombosis within the vessel. The media and internal elastic lamina remain intact.

49 Advanced arteritis There is almost complete destruction of the intima of the vessel, and thrombosis has occurred.

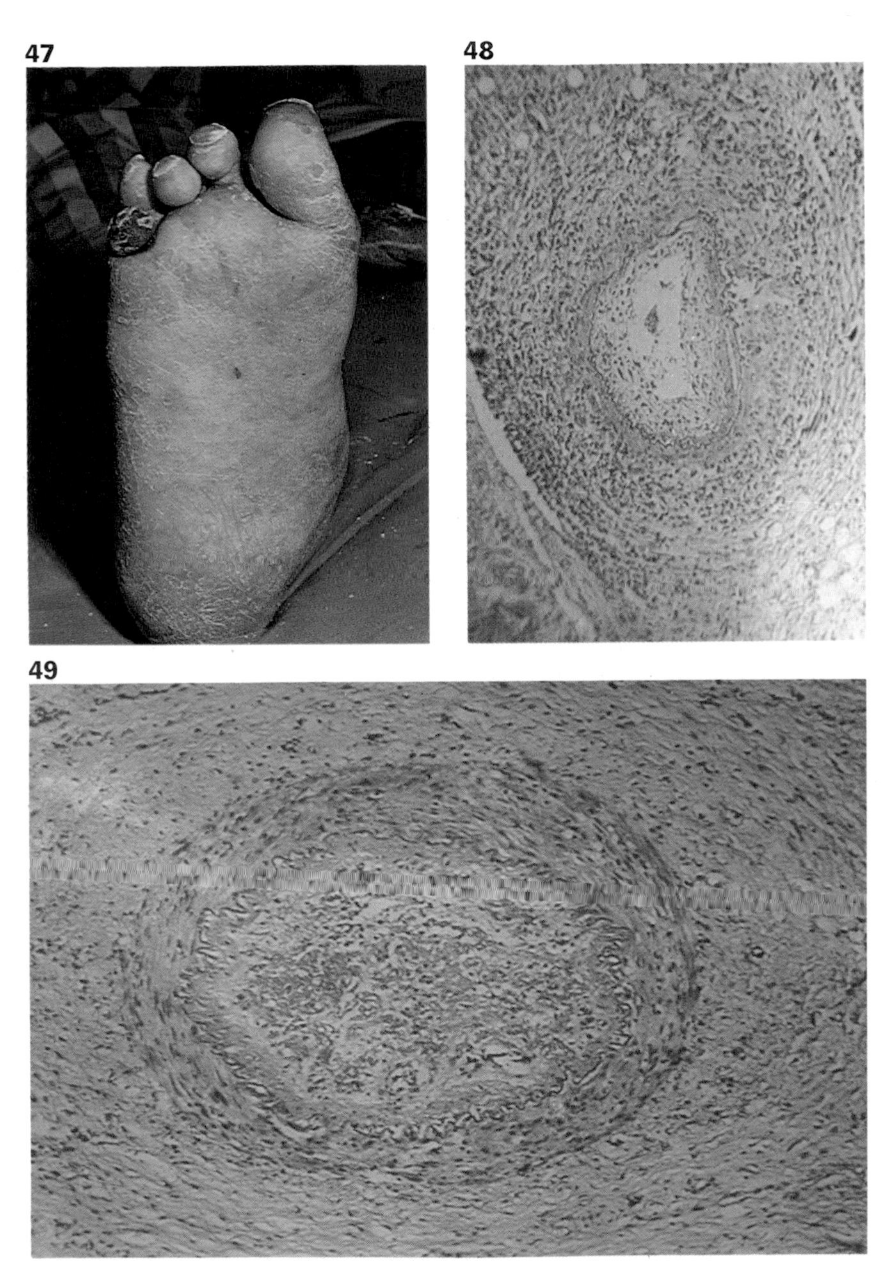
47
48
49

50 Rupture of the sinus of Valsalva, the result of intra-cardiac nodule formation. The patient died suddenly in acute cardiac failure. Clinically, cardiac lesions are rare in rheumatoid arthritis, although valvular lesions and pericarditis are described.

51 ECG of cardiac myopathy Flattening of all waves resembles changes seen in myxoedema. This is another rare condition in rheumatoid arthritis, but may lead to arrhythmias or failure.

52 Renal amyloid The glomerular capillaries are greatly thickened by amyloid deposition. Rheumatoid arthritis is the most important cause of secondary amyloid disease, with an incidence of about 16%. It may present with proteinuria or a nephrotic syndrome. The diagnosis is most readily made by rectal biopsy.

50

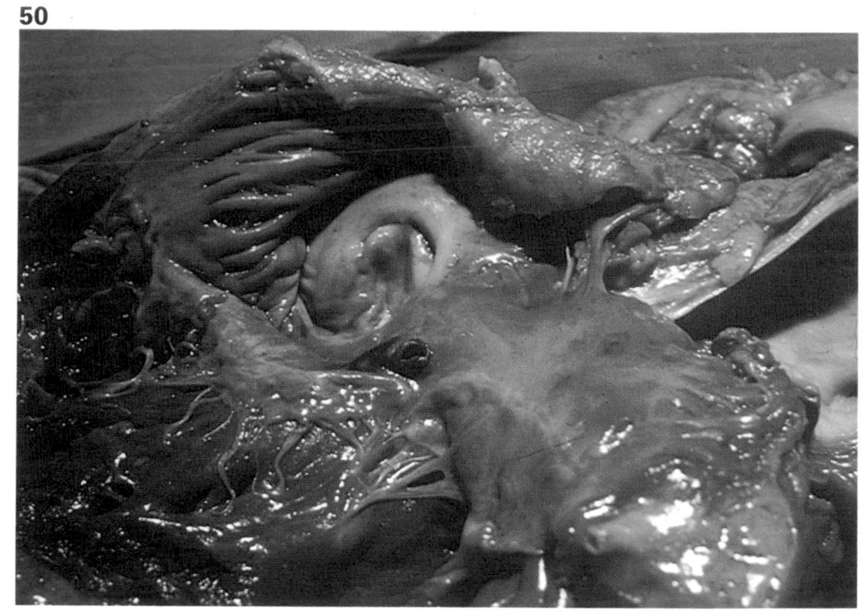

51

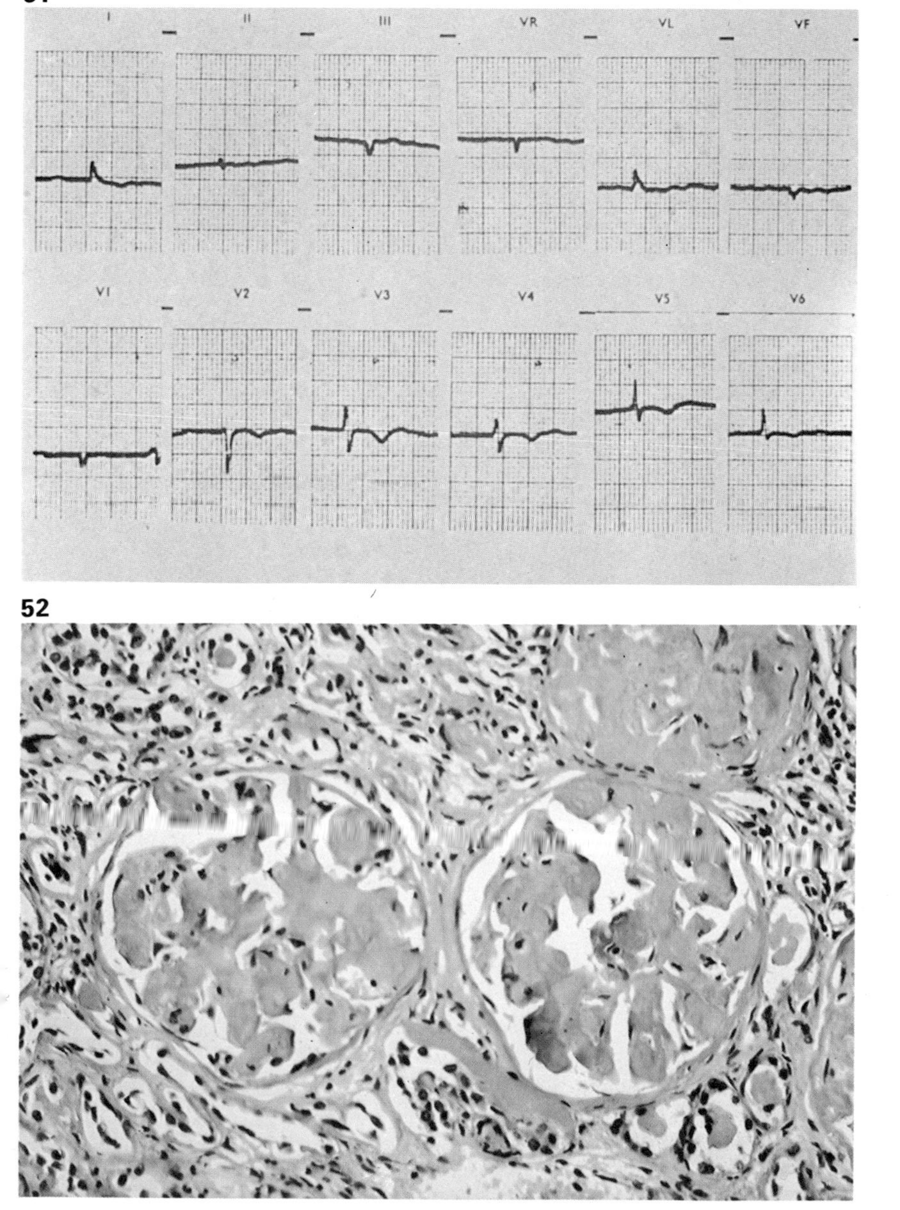

52

NEUROLOGICAL COMPLICATIONS

53 Wasting of the thenar eminences with sensory loss over the median digits is found only in longstanding cases of rheumatoid arthritis. Compression of the median nerve within the carpal tunnel is not uncommon in early stages, and may be bilateral. It is probably due to the increased pressure within the carpus due to inflammation. Another common site of entrapment neuropathy is at the elbow, where the ulnar nerve may be compressed by destructive change within the joint.

54 Peripheral neuropathies The area of sensory loss on the foot and lower leg is shown. The lower limbs are most commonly affected in patients who have evidence of vasculitis. This type of neuropathy may be sensory only with 'stocking' type anaesthesia, or mixed sensori-motor with foot drop.

55 Mixed sensori-motor neuropathy with unilateral foot drop The prognosis in such a patient is generally poor due to the associated vasculitis.

53

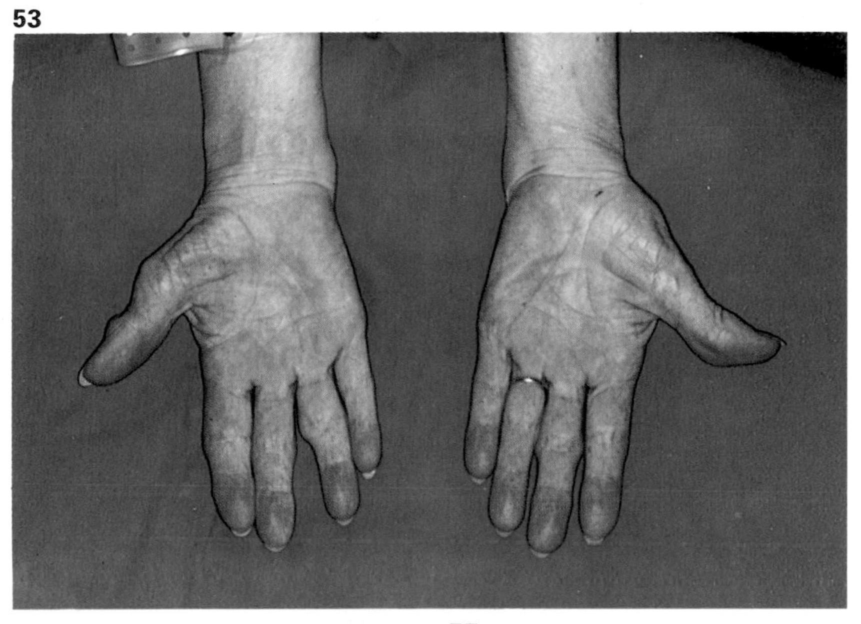

54

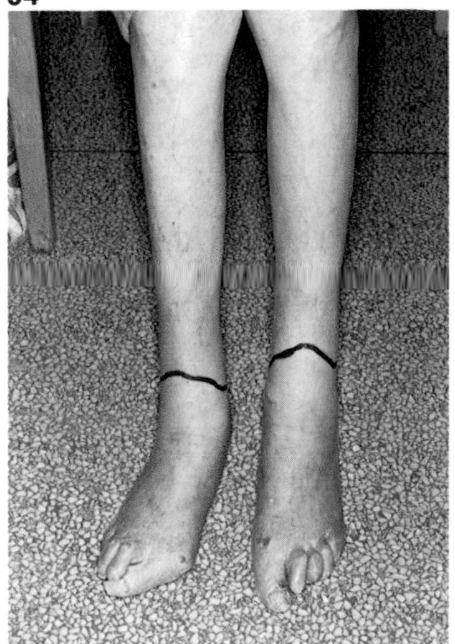

55

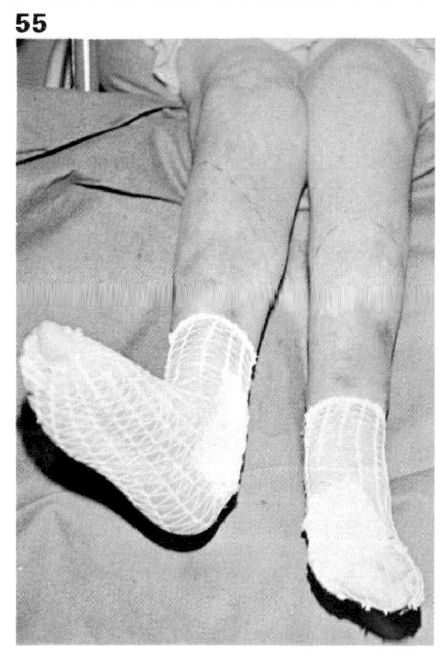

JUVENILE RHEUMATOID ARTHRITIS (STILL'S DISEASE)

This disease differs in certain respects from adult rheumatoid arthritis: (1) the arthritis is generally less destructive, but there is a marked tendency to involvement of the cervical spine; (2) fever, rash, leucocytosis, and lymphadenopathy with splenomegaly are common features; (3) nodules and the presence of rheumatoid factor are far less common than in the adult form of the disease, whereas pericarditis is more frequently seen; (4) iridocyclitis occurs in about 8% of patients, and may be severe, leading to impairment of vision.

A proportion of children suffering from this disease may proceed in later life to develop sacro-iliitis, and this, together with their tendency to the complication of iritis, may in the future influence our classification of the condition, especially as about 29% of such patients have been found to have histo-compatibility antigen HLA-27 (see pages 50 and 51).

56 Growth retardation Because of the inflammatory changes in joints, premature closure of the epiphyses may occur, causing stunting of growth. Treatment with steroids may produce a similar effect. The girl on the left developed juvenile rheumatoid arthritis at the age of eight, from which time she was treated with steroids. Both girls are in their early twenties.

57 Band keratopathy resulting from severe iridocyclitis in juvenile rheumatoid arthritis.

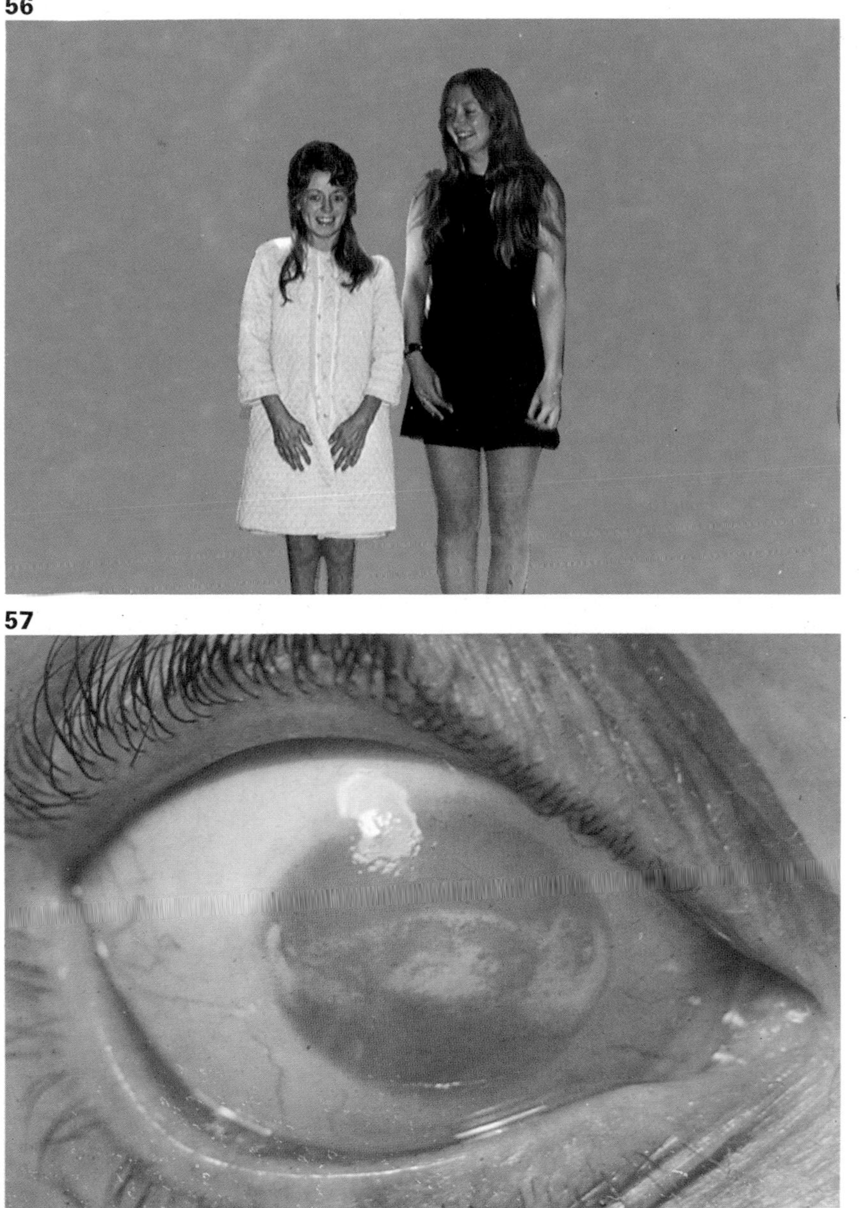

56

57

Sero-negative Spondarthritides

This title is used to describe four diseases (psoriatic arthritis, Reiter's syndrome, ankylosing spondylitis, and enteropathic arthritis) which, although in some ways resembling rheumatoid arthritis, exhibit certain important differences. In particular, all show a negative test for rheumatoid factor, and in each there is a tendency to involvement of the sacro-iliac joints and spine. Other overlapping features include the occurrence of uveitis, absence of subcutaneous nodules, the similarity of the skin and nail changes in psoriatic arthritis and Reiter's syndrome, and the occasional occurrence of aortitis in ankylosing spondylitis and Reiter's syndrome. Histo-compatibility antigen HLA–27 occurs in all these diseases in a higher percentage than in the normal population (about 8%).

Psoriatic arthritis Psoriasis is a common skin disease, often hereditary, and affecting up to 2% of the population. About 8% of those suffering psoriasis develop an arthritis which differs from rheumatoid arthritis in a number of ways:

1. There is no female preponderance.
2. Rheumatoid factor and subcutaneous nodules are absent.
3. Joint involvement tends to be asymmetrical and may affect the terminal interphalangeal joints and sacro-iliac joints.
4. Skin and joint lesions tend to remit and relapse synchronously.
5. HLA–27 is found in about 18% of patients with only peripheral joint involvement; if the sacro-iliac joints are involved, this rises to 35%.

Reiter's syndrome The disease is almost confined to males and is usually sexually transmitted, but may follow epidemic dysentery. A family history of psoriasis is more common in those suffering the disease than in the normal population. The classical triad of urethritis, arthritis, and conjunctivitis is not always complete, conjunctivitis occurring in only 60% of cases. The following are its main features:

1. Genito-urinary involvement: non-specific urethritis, prostatitis, or haemorrhagic cystitis.
2. An inflammatory arthritis predominantly involving the weight-bearing joints (toes, ankles or knees), and often followed by sacro-iliitis with para-spinal ligamentous calcification or ossification.

3. Ocular lesions: conjunctivitis in the early stage, iritis later affecting 10% of patients.
4. Mucosal lesions: shallow penile ulceration, circinate balanitis, and ulceration of the buccal mucosa and tongue.
5. Skin and nail lesions: keratodermia blennorrhagica which may be indistinguishable histologically from pustular psoriasis, and nail dystrophy also closely resembling that seen in psoriasis.
6. Cardiac involvement: rarely aortitis or pericarditis.
7. HLA–27 is positive in about 70% of cases.

Ankylosing spondylitis Heredity appears to play some part in the aetiology of ankylosing spondylitis, the disease appearing 30 times more commonly in relatives of sufferers than in non-spondylitic controls.
Its main features are:

1. A marked male predominance with onset in the late 'teens or early twenties.
2. Bilateral sacro-iliitis usually proceeding to para-spinal ligamentous calcification or ossification with ankylosis of the spinal facet joints.
3. Peripheral joint involvement more common in the hips and shoulders than elsewhere.
4. A high incidence (about 25%) of iritis.
5. Rarely aortitis or pulmonary fibrosis affecting the upper lung fields.
6. In this disease HLA–27 is positive in over 90% of patients.

Enteropathic arthritis Arthritis may complicate ulcerative colitis, Crohn's disease (regional enteritis), or Whipple's disease. For practical purposes the forms of arthritis which occur in ulcerative colitis and Crohn's disease are similar and may be considered together. There appear to be two quite distinct entities:

1. A peripheral arthritis occurring in between 10–20% of patients, and with a close temporal relation to the activity of the bowel disease. Lower limb joints, particularly knees and ankles, are involved more commonly than others, and the arthritis tends to be transitory and to flit from joint to joint. Cure of the bowel disease leads to remission of the arthritis.
2. Sacro-iliitis which may proceed to spinal ligamentous calcification or ossification, giving a clinical and radiological picture indistinguishable from ankylosing spondylitis. Unlike the peripheral arthritis there is no temporal relation to the bowel disease, nor does treatment of the latter affect the course of the spondylitis.
3. In the presence of sacro-iliitis HLA–27 positivity amounts to about 67%, but if peripheral arthritis occurs alone, positivity is no more than in the normal population.

PSORIATIC ARTHRITIS

Arthritis occurs in about 8% of patients who have psoriasis. The arthritis differs from true rheumatoid arthritis in several ways: (1) terminal interphalangeal joints may be affected, and sacro-iliitis with calcification of paraspinal ligaments may occur; (2) skin nodules are absent; (3) tests for rheumatoid factor are negative; (4) there is no female predominance.

58 Early psoriasis of the nails (**'thimble pitting'**) is well marked. (*Picture by kind permission of Dr G M Levene, St John's Hospital, London*)

59 Advanced nail psoriasis shows dystrophy of the nails, discoloration and sub-ungual separation. Note the redness and swelling of several terminal interphalangeal joints associated with the neighbouring nail dystrophy.

It would seem that nail involvement in some way enhances liability to develop arthropathy, since 80% of patients with psoriatic arthritis have both skin and nail lesions.

58

59

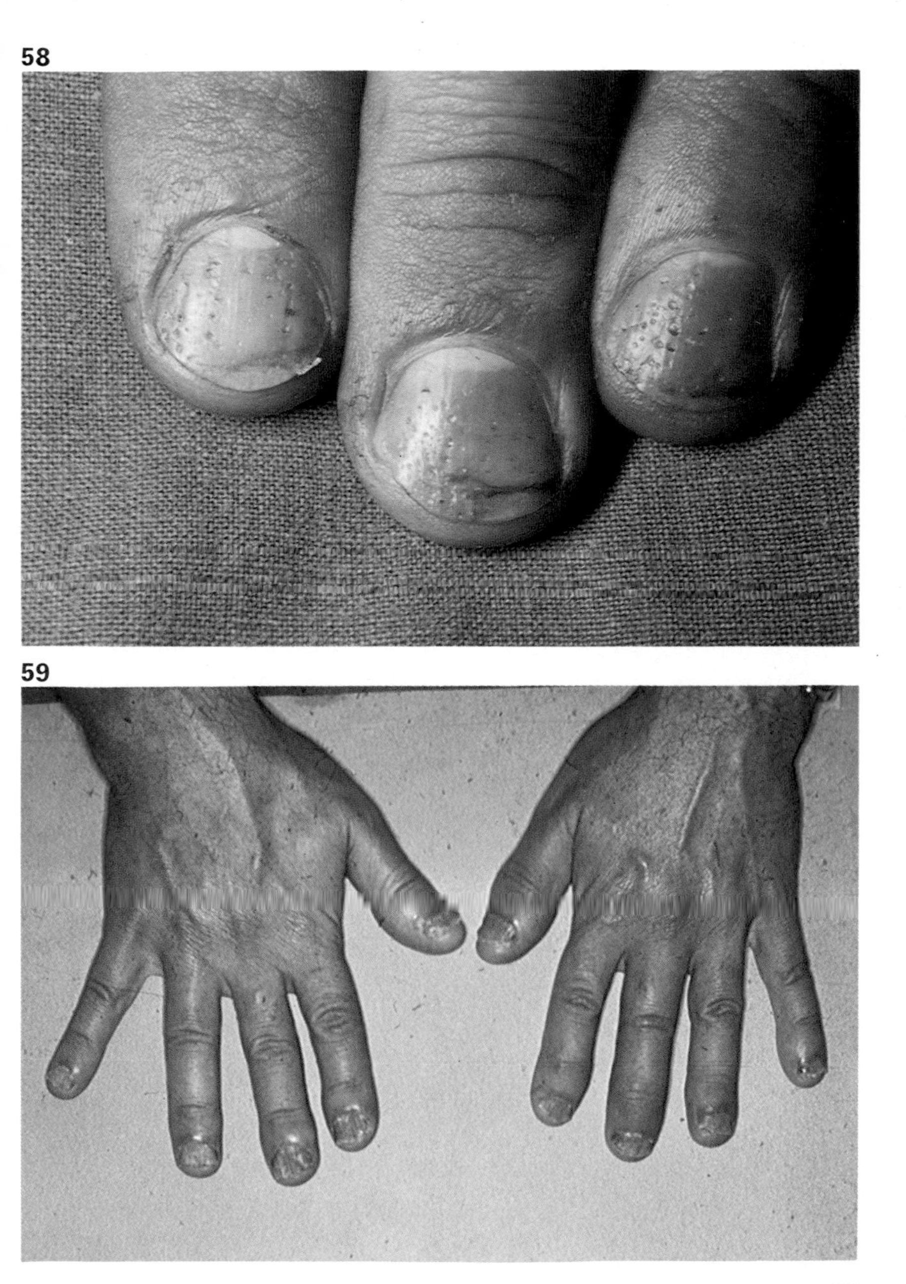

60 More advanced psoriatic arthritis of the hands Note changes in the metacarpophalangeal and interphalangeal joints which closely resemble rheumatoid arthritis, but again the terminal interphalangeal joints are affected.

61 X-ray of early psoriatic arthritis Note erosive changes in the left ring and right little finger terminal interphalangeal joints. Cartilage loss and erosions in other joints resemble changes seen in rheumatoid arthritis.

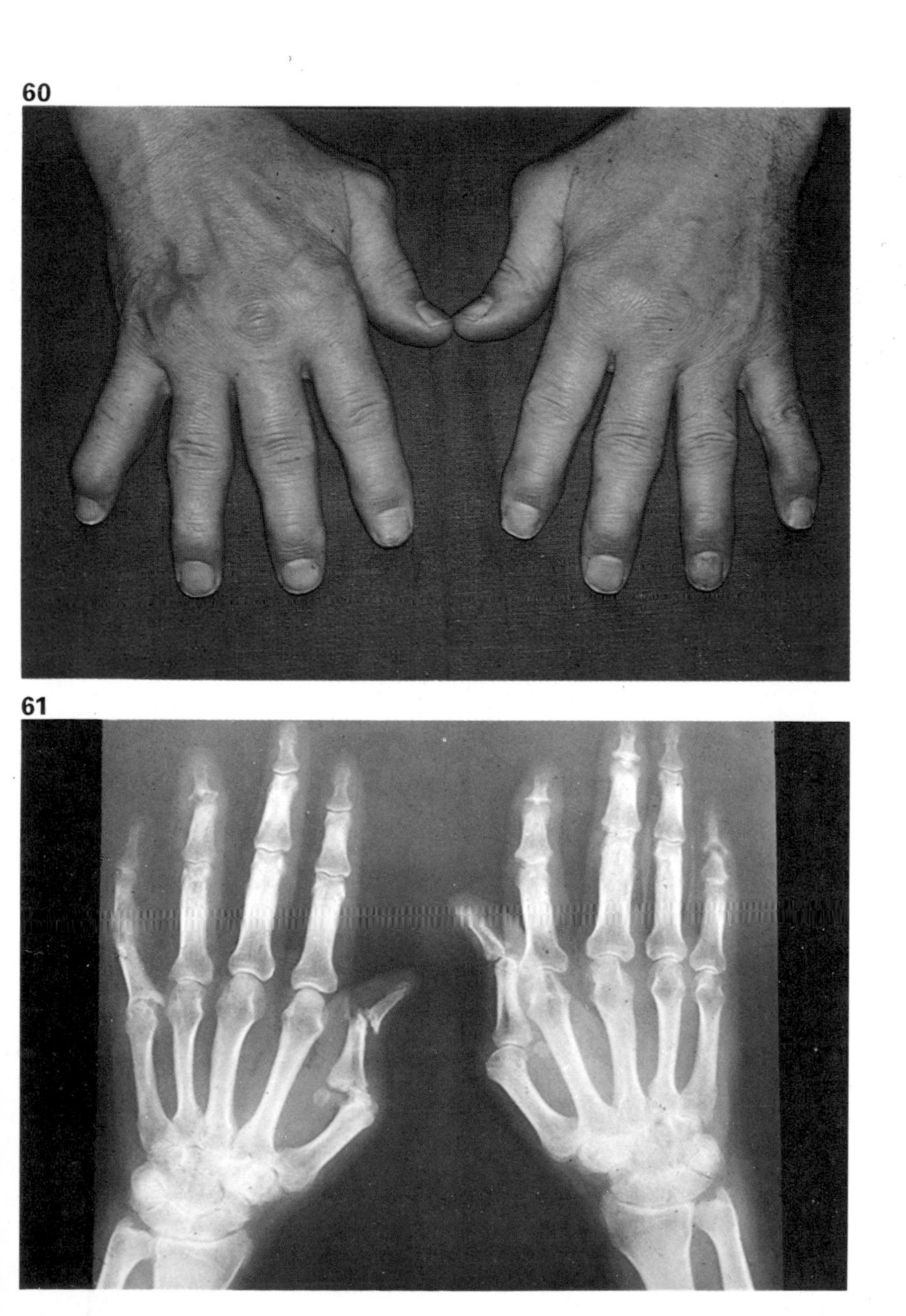
60
61

62 X-ray of advanced psoriatic arthritis Changes are often grossly destructive with subluxation or ankylosis. Whittling down of the phalanges as seen here in the thumb is characteristic.

63 Typical psoriasis involving the trunk

64 Bilateral sacro-iliitis occurs in 10–30% of patients with psoriatic arthritis. This is sometimes followed by paraspinal ligamentous calcification or ossification resembling ankylosing spondylitis.

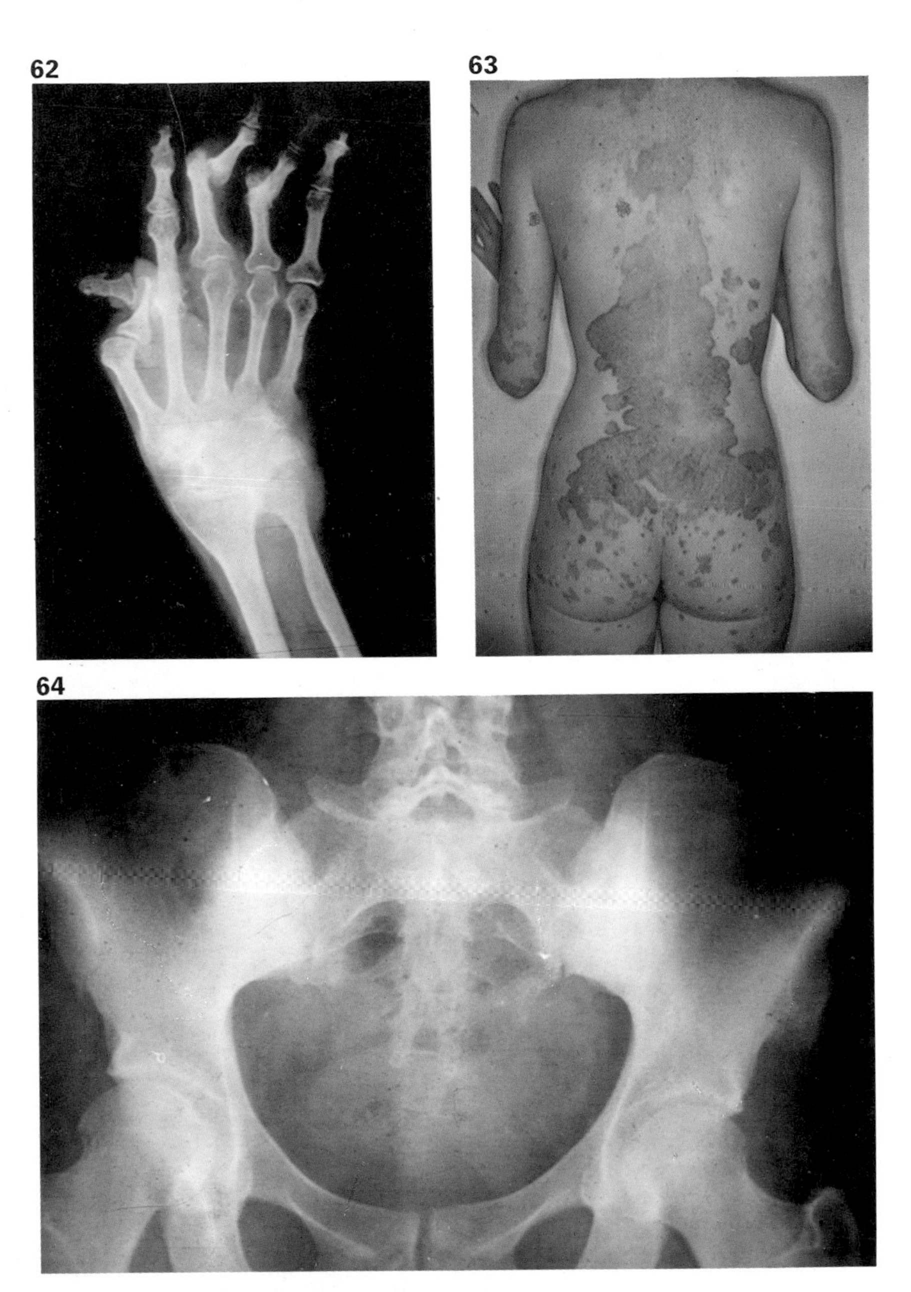
62
63
64

REITER'S SYNDROME

The classical triad in this disease is non-specific urethritis, arthritis, and conjunctivitis. Arthritis usually follows the urethritis after an interval of 1–3 weeks, and in the early stages is nearly always confined to the joints of the lower limb, particularly the small joints of the toes and ankles. The urethritis may be transient and overlooked by the physician, or concealed by the patient, who may be too worried or ashamed to reveal it. Prostatitis should be looked for, and the secretion examined after prostatic massage. In the same way, the conjunctivitis may be so transient as to be forgotten by the patient. However, suspicion of the diagnosis should be aroused if the patient is a young male with an acute mono- or polyarthritis affecting the feet, ankles or knees.

65 Acute Reiter's syndrome There is marked swelling and redness of the small joints of the toes of the left foot, and destructive changes have shortened the great toe. Note the similarity of the skin lesions (keratodermia blennorrhagica) to pustular psoriasis, and of the nail lesions to those of advanced psoriasis. In Reiter's syndrome one or more of the nails may be completely shed.

66 Periostitis over lower end of both medial malleoli X-ray changes may show osteoporosis around affected joints, which may later proceed to erosion and destructive changes as seen in other inflammatory arthritides. Periostitis around affected joints is typical.

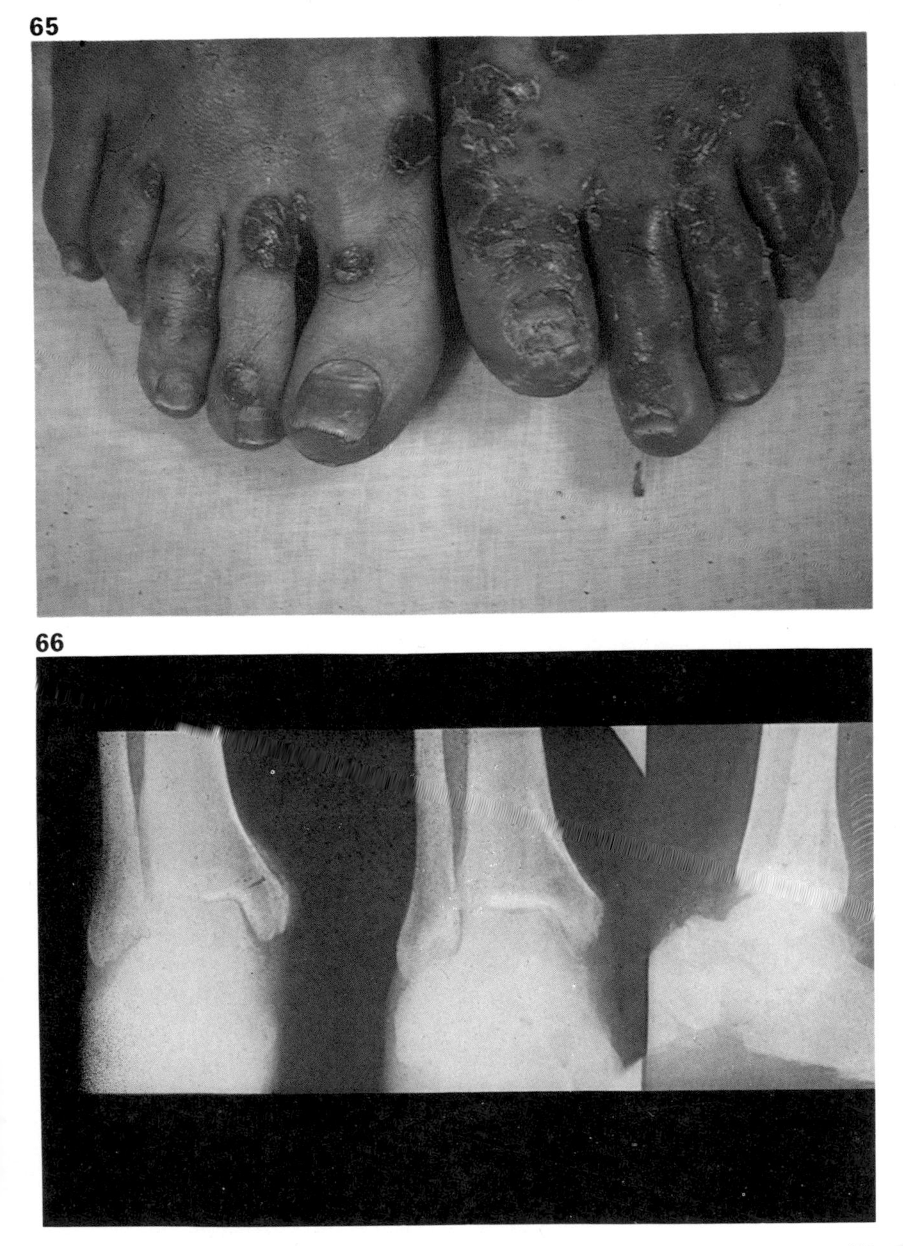

67 Painful heel is a common symptom X-ray may show calcaneal spurring and sometimes erosion of the os calcis.

68 Keratodermia blennorrhagica occurs in the more severe relapsing cases, and is often confined to the feet and lower legs. Both clinically and histologically, these skin lesions closely resemble pustular psoriasis.

69 Advanced keratodermia blennorrhagica of the feet and lower legs

67

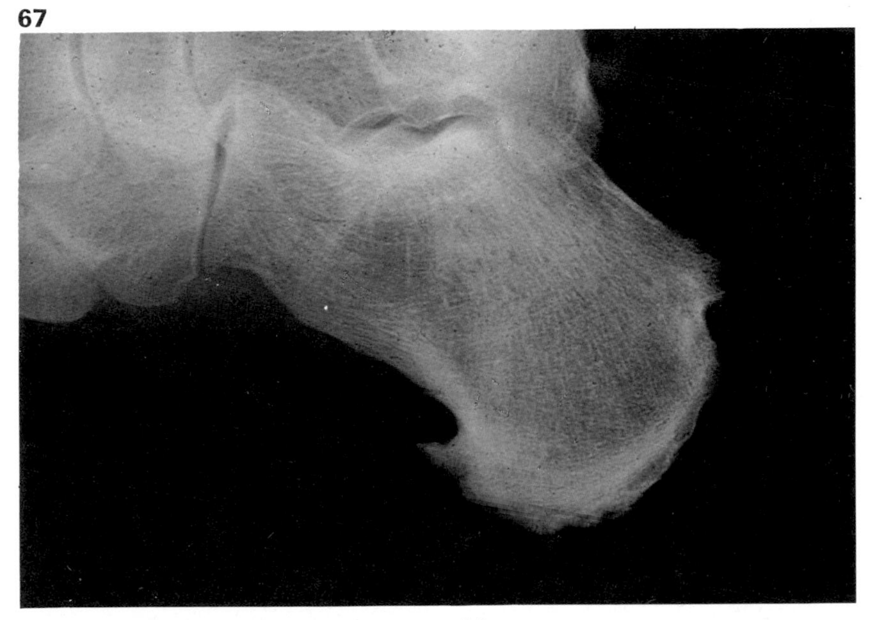

68

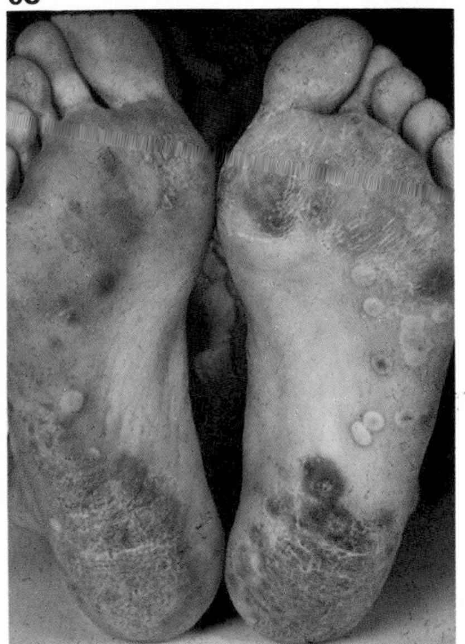

69

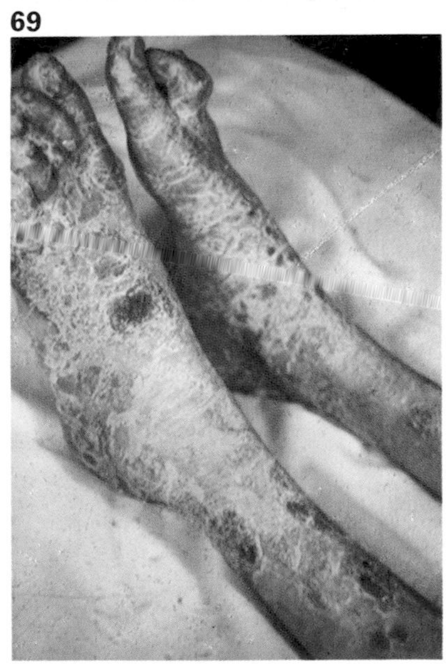

70 The hands in advanced Reiter's syndrome Note that the nail changes and involvement of the terminal interphalangeal joints bear a close resemblance to psoriatic arthritis.

71 Nail dystrophy in the toes in Reiter's syndrome Again note the close resemblance to psoriatic nail dystrophy.

72 Balanitis of the penis Superficial ulceration of mucous membranes occurs in the more severe type of case. Similar changes may affect the buccal mucosa. Ulcers around the penile meatus are also characteristic.

70

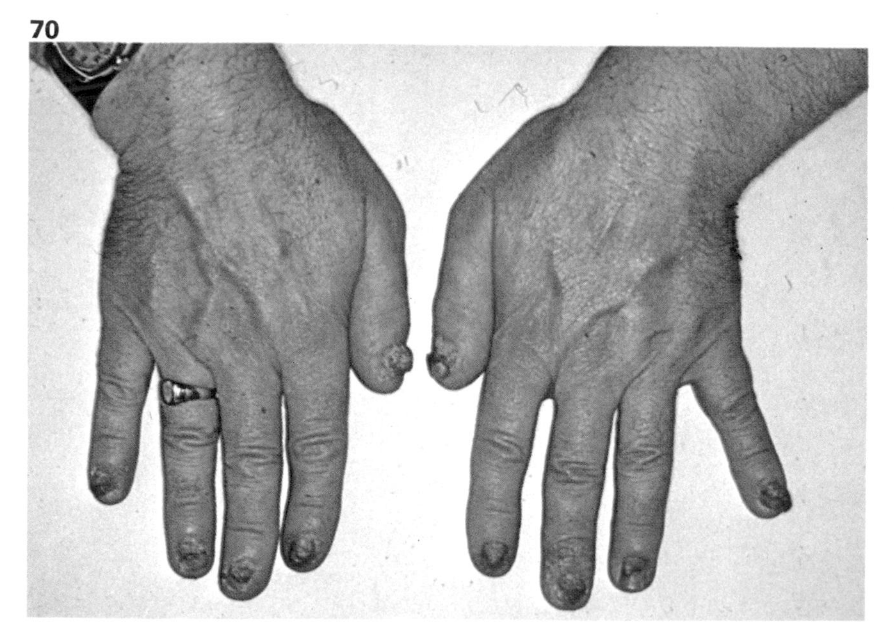

71

72

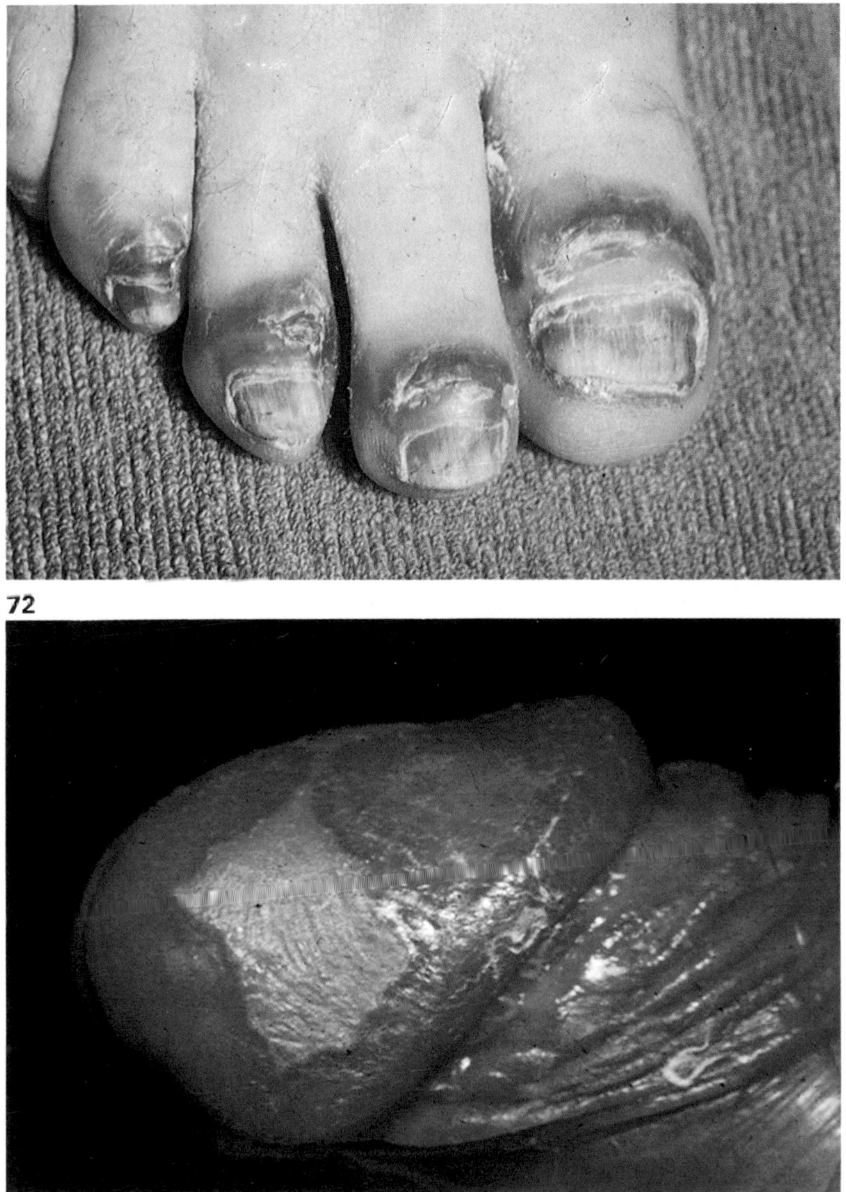

73 Conjunctivitis is not an essential part of the triad of Reiter's syndrome, as it may be absent in up to 40% of cases. It is always bilateral, and may be transient and missed by the clinician.

74 Sacro-iliitis may occur, as in psoriatic arthritis, and proceed to paraspinal ligamentous calcification and ossification, giving a final picture which closely resembles ankylosing spondylitis.

75 Acute iritis develops in 20% of patients with Reiter's syndrome, and is usually associated with severe and relapsing disease.

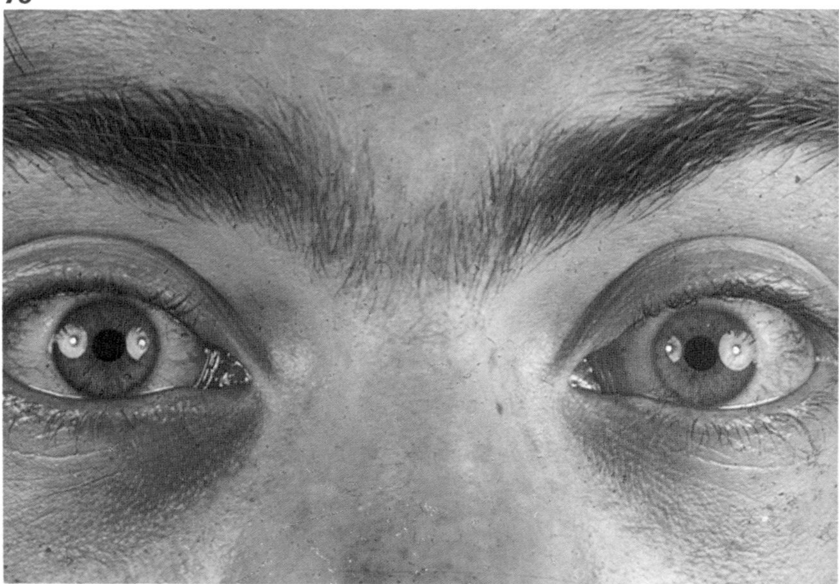

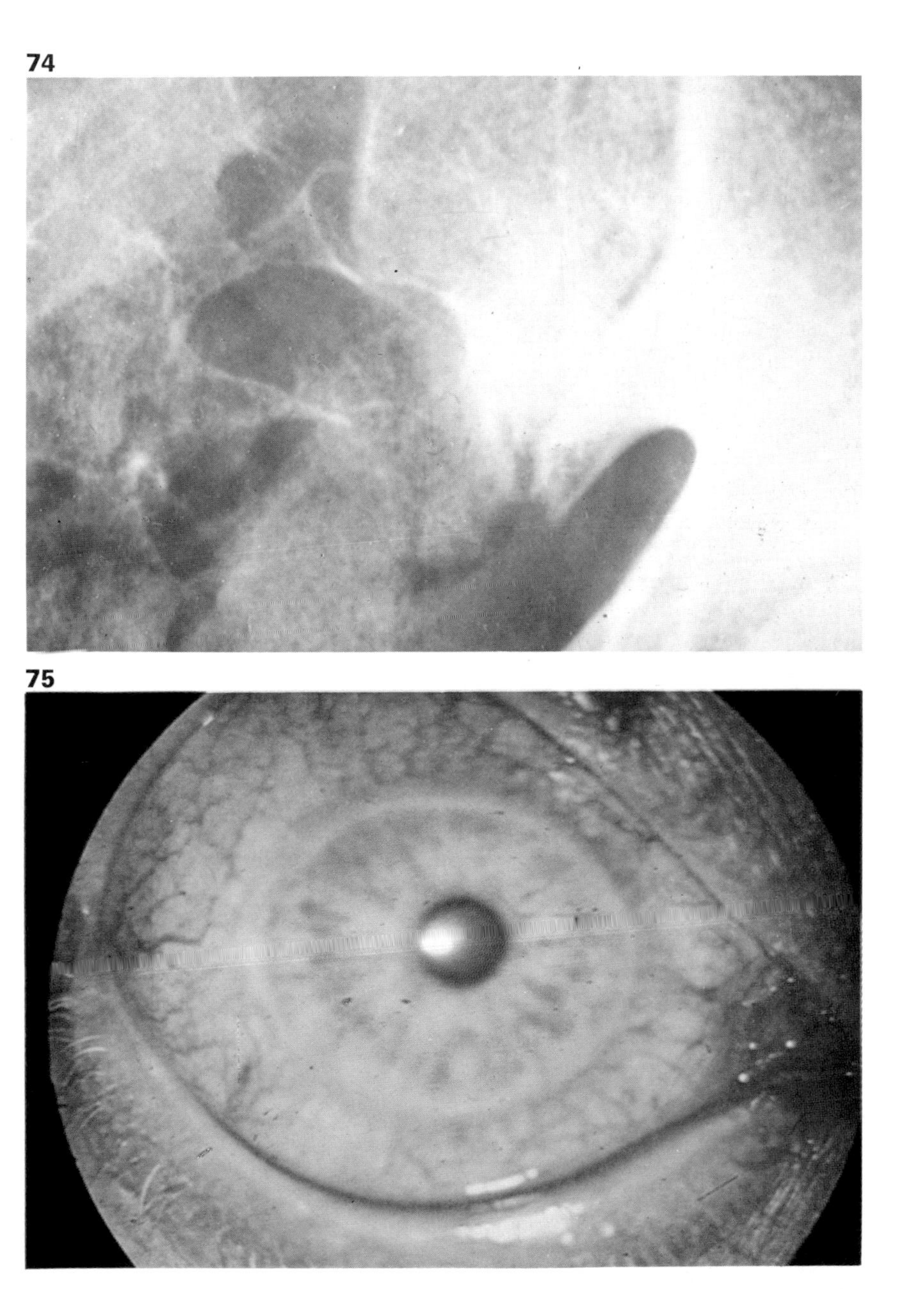

74

75

ANKYLOSING SPONDYLITIS

This disease is much more common in men than in women (ratio 8 :1), and symptoms are usually noticed in the late teens or early twenties, with increasing aching and stiffness in the lower back. Many cases remain mild and almost non-progressive while others exhibit a gradual advance of the disease up the spine with progressive spinal ligamentous calcification and ossification which may result in total rigidity of the entire spinal column. Involvement of the hip and shoulder joints is not uncommon, but other peripheral joints are rarely involved, nodules are absent, and tests for rheumatoid factor are usually negative.

76 Typical kyphosis

77 Posterior view of the same patient

78 Forward flexion is achieved by movement of the hip joints. The lumbar and dorsal spines are totally stiff.

79 Limitation of side flexion is an early sign and will often distinguish the disease from mechanical derangements of the spine, in which side flexion is usually remarkably free and painless.

76

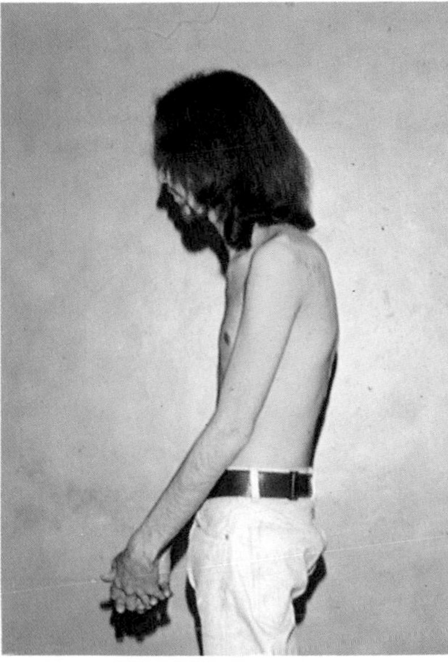

77

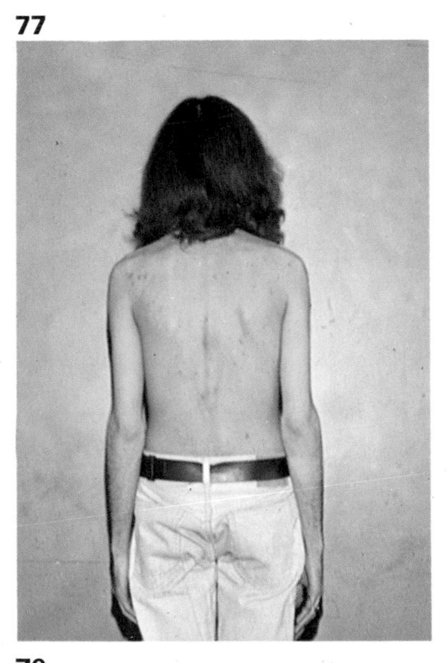

78

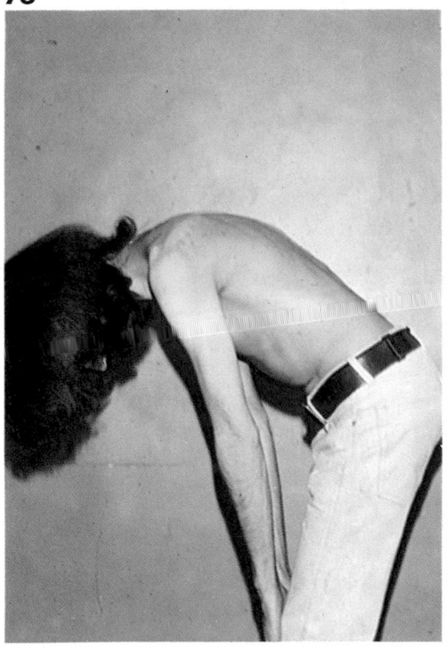

79

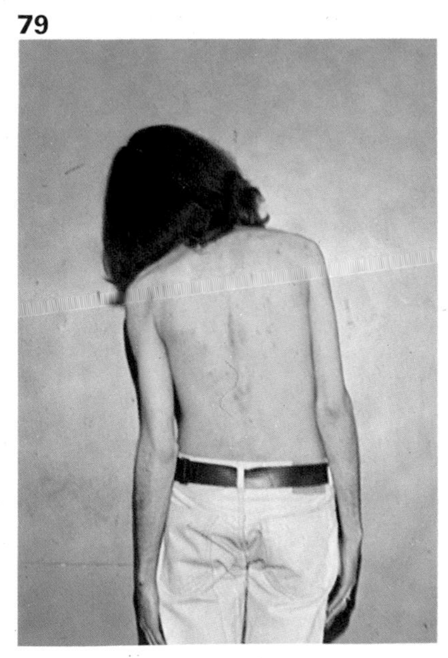

80 Radiograph of the sacro-iliac joints shows erosions and sclerosis of the margins of the joints (as seen in the right joint), proceeding to ankylosis (as seen in the lower pole of the left joint). Note also erosion of the symphysis pubis. A fluffy periosteal reaction is often also seen at the site of muscle attachments, particularly around the illiac crests.

81 Late x-ray changes in ankylosing spondylitis The sacro-iliac joints are obliterated by ankylosis, and ossification has occurred in the para-spinal ligaments. Note also affection of the hip joints.

80

81

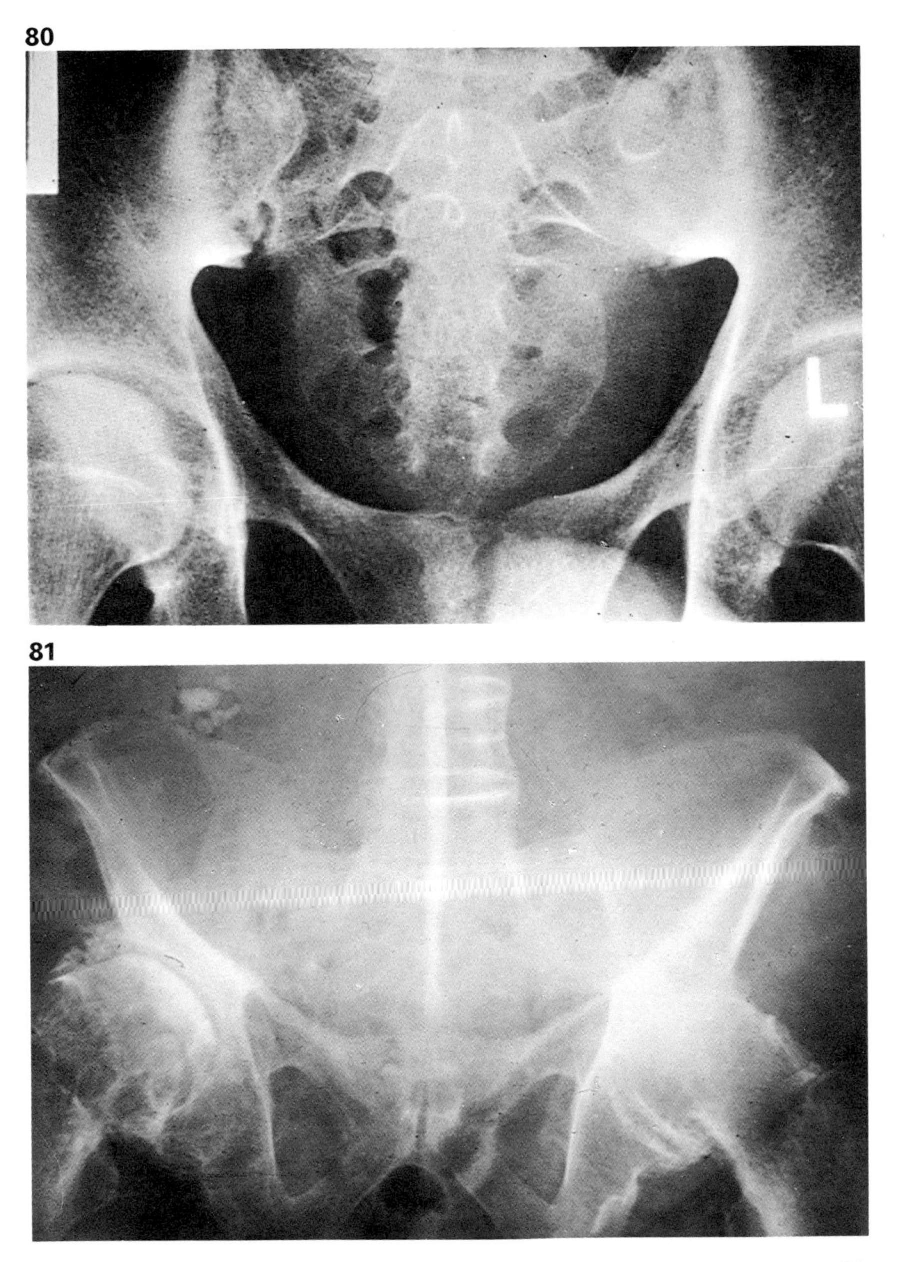

82 Lateral view of the lumbar spine Ossification of anterior spinal ligament can be seen.

83 Antero-posterior view of the upper lumbar spine shows calcification in the lateral spinal ligaments.

84 The cervical spine in ankylosing spondylitis Again there is calcification of the anterior spinal ligament.

Atlanto-axial subluxation may occur in the cervical spine affected by ankylosing spondylitis as it does in rheumatoid arthritis, but subluxation at lower levels rarely if ever occurs, presumably because the vertebrae are splinted by the ossified ligaments. Due to its rigidity, however, the cervical spine is unduly susceptible to trauma, and fracture may occur following relatively trivial injury.

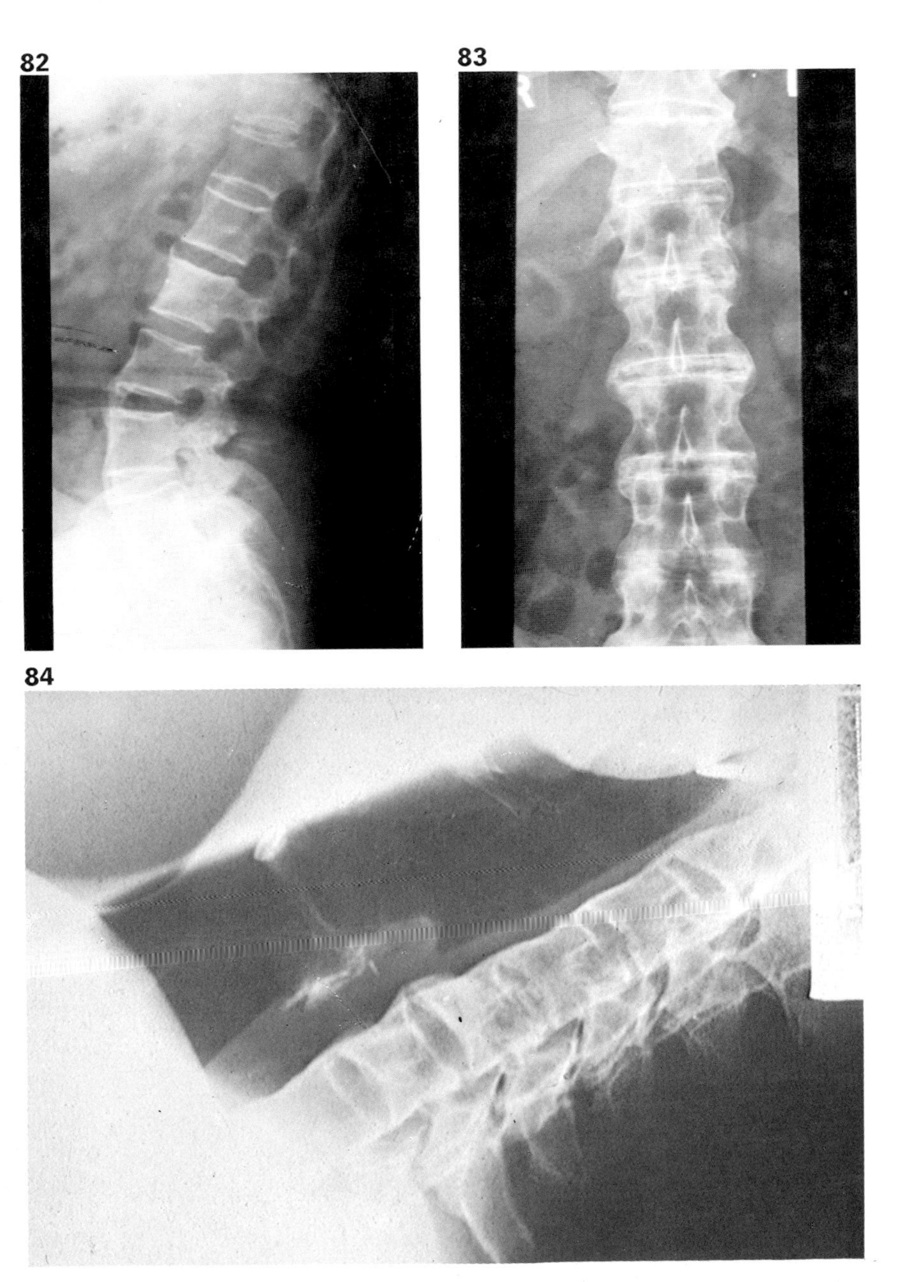

85 Acute iritis is the commonest complication of ankylosing spondylitis and occurs in about 25% of patients.

86 Posterior synechiae with permanent damage to vision often develop as a result of repeated attacks of iritis.

85

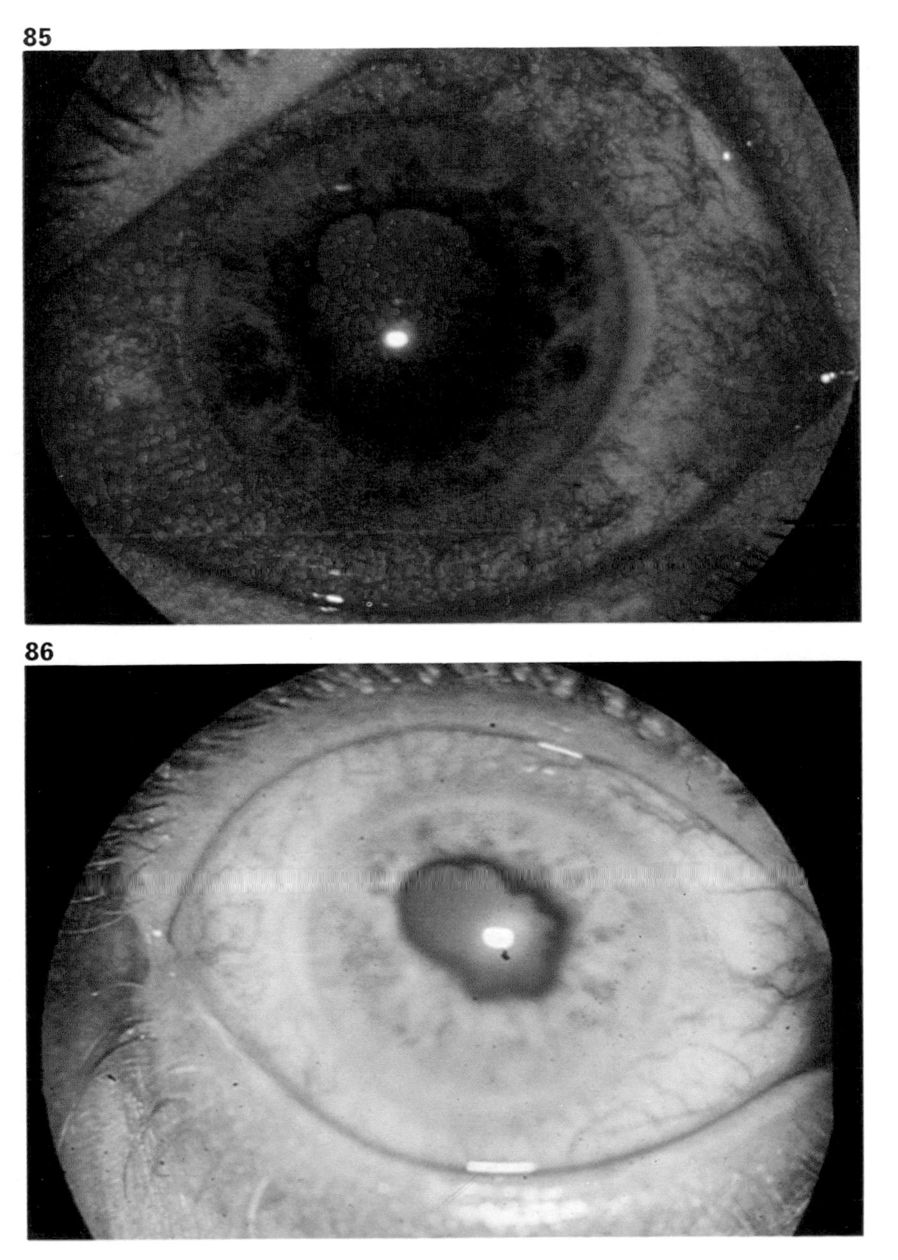

86

ENTEROPATHIC ARTHRITIS

This may present as a complication of ulcerative colitis, Crohn's disease (regional ileitis), or Whipple's disease. All these bowel diseases may be associated with sacro-iliitis and para-spinal ligamentous calcification. A peripheral arthritis may also occur, usually predominantly affecting the joints of the lower limb.

87 Ulcerative colitis and effusion into both knees The latter cleared up when the colitis was successfully treated.

Unlike the peripheral arthritis, sacro-iliitis and spondylitis bear no temporal relationship to the bowel disease, nor is their course affected by successful treatment of the bowel.

87

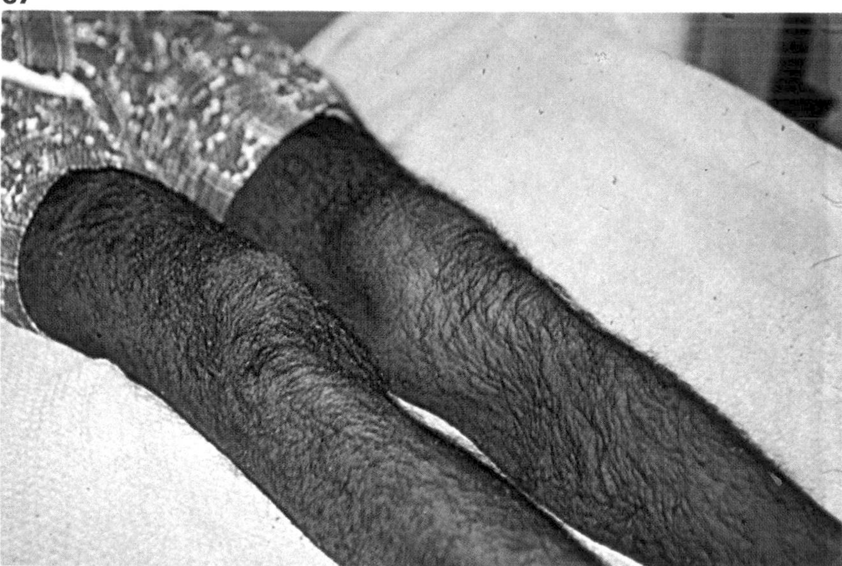

Degenerative Joint Disease

Affection of synovial joints by degenerative processes is now generally known as osteoarthrosis (formerly osteoarthritis). Degeneration of intervertebral discs, which are fibro-cartilaginous joints (synchondroses), is known as spondylosis.

Osteoarthrosis Although primarily considered to be part of the ageing process, osteoarthrosis appears to have a number of factors in its aetiology. There is evidence of a genetic determinant, but in addition, occupation, obesity, or previous injury to the joint may determine its site and severity.

The major lesion in affected joints is in articular cartilage, which shows softening, fibrillation and flaking. The underlying causes of these changes are still obscure, but it would seem that both mechanical and biochemical factors play a part. Subchondral bone undergoes thickening and sclerosis, and cysts may occur in deeper layers, perhaps due to herniation of synovial fluid through breaks in the trabeculae. Osteophyte formation at the margin of affected joints is characteristic.

In general, osteoarthritis may be distinguished from rheumatoid arthritis by the absence of signs of inflammation in affected joints and of a disturbance of general health, together with the finding of a normal E.S.R. and negative tests for rheumatoid factor. Radiological changes do not necessarily mirror the symptomatology. Disability is usually not serious unless the hip joints are affected.

Spondylosis Degeneration of intervertebral discs may be accompanied by osteoarthrosis of the diarthrodial (facet) joints. Radiological changes of disc degeneration are almost universal in the older age group but do not necessarily indicate that they are the cause of local pain and stiffness. As with osteoarthrosis of peripheral joints, spondylosis rarely causes major disability, but advanced changes in the cervical region of the spine may result in local compression of the spinal cord giving rise to long tract signs – usually a spastic quadriplegia.

OSTEOARTHROSIS

88 Heberden's nodes (involvement of the terminal interphalangeal joints) are the most characteristic features of osteoarthrosis of the finger joints. Note early involvement of both thumbs, and the right middle and both little fingers. Advanced changes with deformity affect the left index and middle fingers.

89 X-ray of hands with Heberden's nodes Cartilage thinning, osteophyte formation, and sub-chondral bone sclerosis affect many of the terminal interphalangeal joints. Changes are also present in some of the proximal interphalangeal joints.

90 Osteoarthrosis of the first carpometacarpal joint is common and may affect grip. Large osteophytes are present around the joint.

88

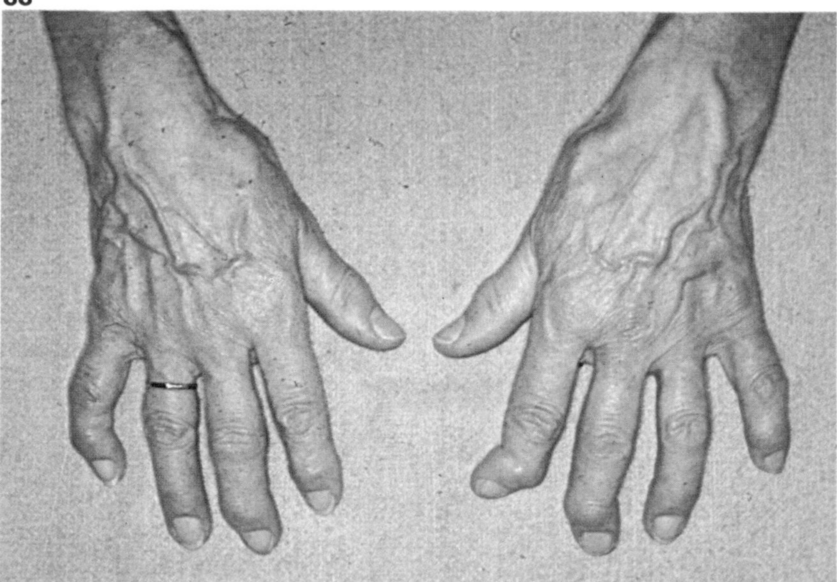

89

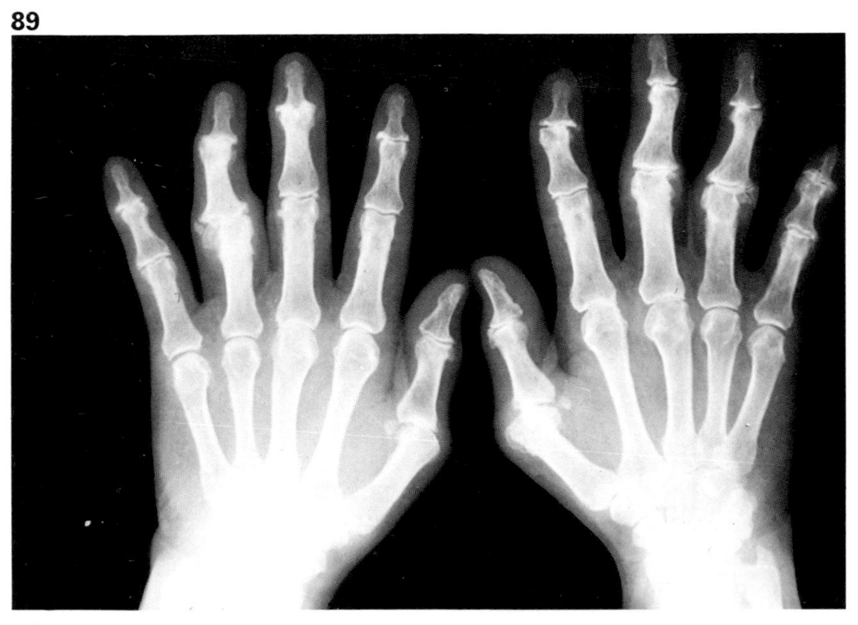

90

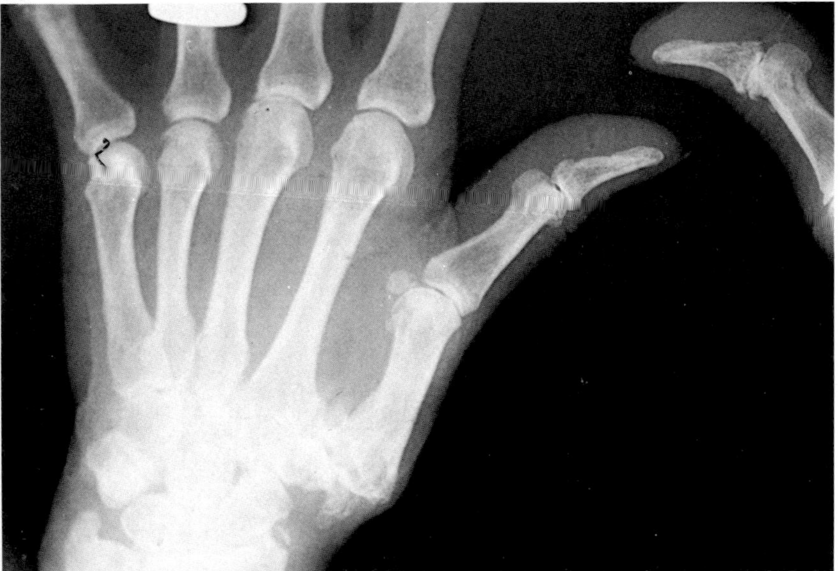

91 & 92 Osteoarthrosis of the knee In the early stage (top left) there is some cartilage loss in the medial compartment with small osteophytes on the medial margins of the femoral condyle and tibial plateau. At a more advanced stage (top right) changes extend to both compartments of the knee.

93 Lateral x-ray of early osteoarthrosis of the knee Note involvement of patello-femoral joint with osteophytosis.

94 Severe osteoarthrosis of the knee with gross involvement of patello-femoral joint. In such cases loose bodies – either single or multiple – are not uncommon, but rarely seem to cause mechanical locking of the joint.

91

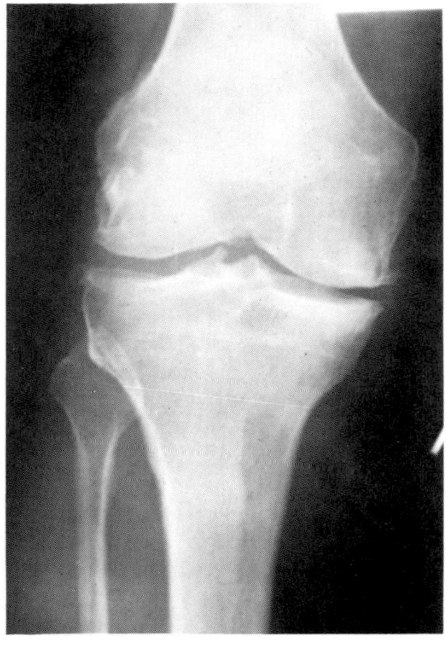

92

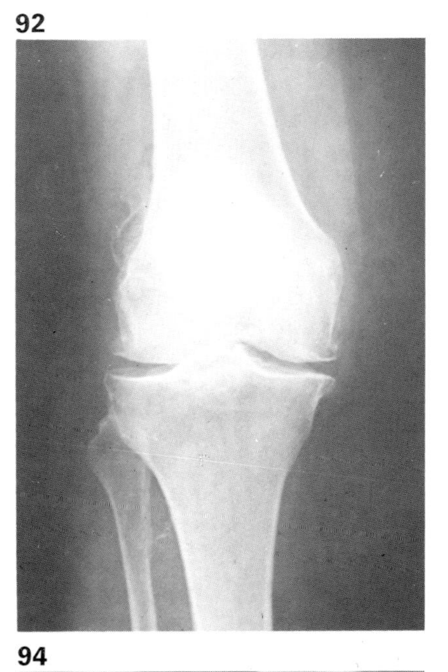

93

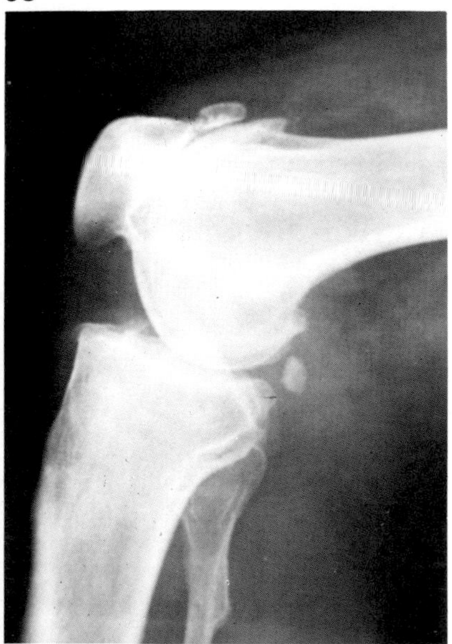

94

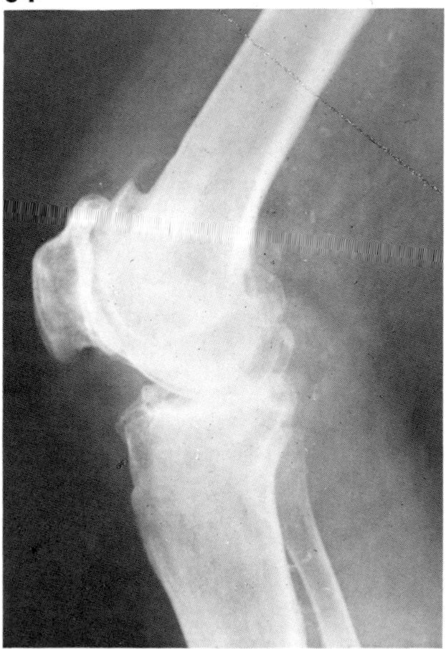

95 Early bilateral osteoarthrosis of the hip joints In the left hip there is generalized narrowing of the joint space. In addition, the right hip shows osteophyte formation at the margins of the femoral head.

96 Osteoarthrosis of the shoulder shows cartilage loss, subchondral bone sclerosis, and osteophytes on the humeral head. Apart from the hands, knees, and hips, osteoarthrosis of other peripheral joints is relatively uncommon, but radiological changes show the same signs.

95

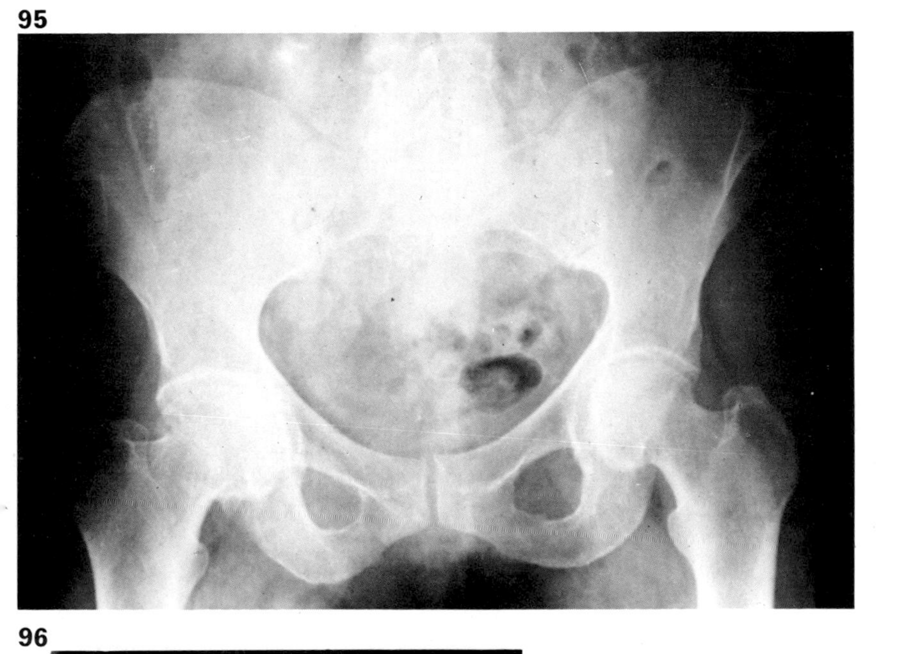

96

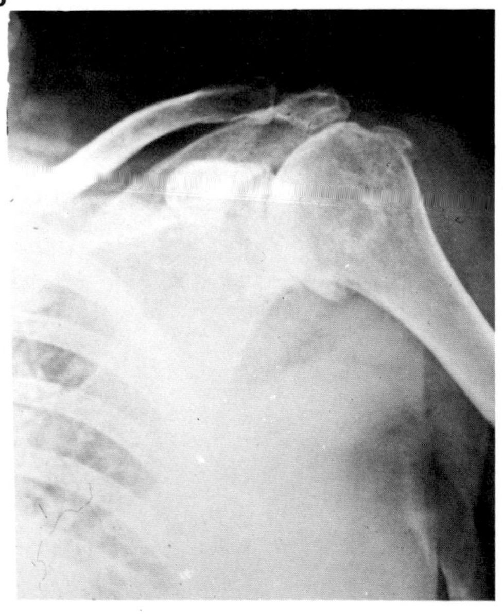

SPONDYLOSIS

97 Early degenerative arthritis of the cervical spine (cervical spondylosis) Note narrowing of C.5–6 disc with osteophytes on anterior border of adjacent vertebrae.

98 Advanced cervical spondylosis Generalized disc degeneration has occurred. In the presence of cervical stenosis, cord compression may occur, giving rise to long tract signs involving the lateral and posterior columns.

99 Dorsal spondylosis Large osteophytes in the lower dorsal segment have fused.

100 Lumbar spondylosis There is generalized disc degeneration and osteophytes.

97

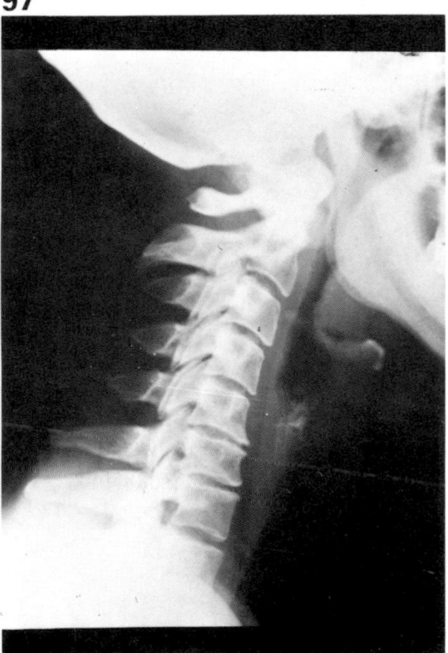

98

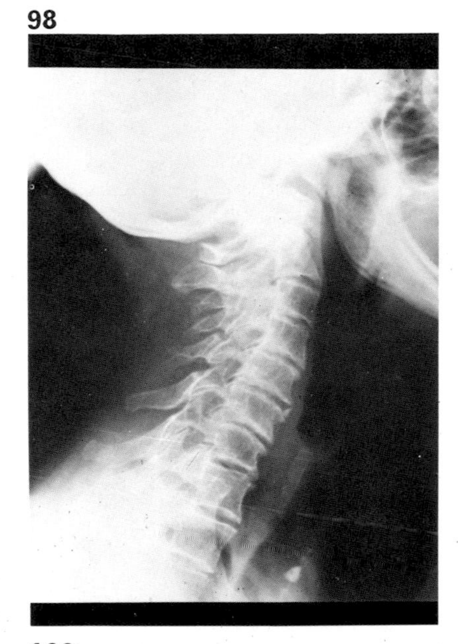

99

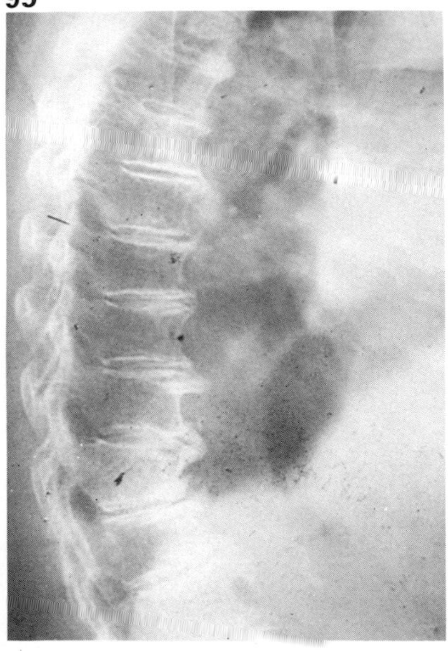

100

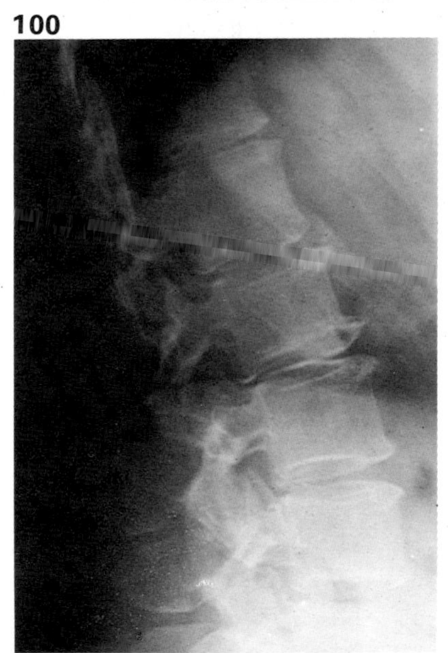

Crystal Synovitis

There are two common forms of crystal-induced synovitis: gout and chondrocalcinosis (pseudo-gout or calcium gout).

Gout may be primary with a positive family history of 60% of cases, or secondary to other diseases, e.g. the myeloproliferative disorders or renal failure. Certain drugs may also cause hyperuricaemia such as a low dosage of salicylates or the thiazide diuretics.

Acute gout most commonly affects the metatarsophalangeal joint of the great toe, although any joint may be so affected. Pain is usually much more severe than in other types of inflammatory arthritis, but even if left untreated the attack will almost always subside within 2–3 weeks. Repeated attacks of gout over many years may lead to tophaceous deposits around affected joints or in cartilage (e.g. the ear). If untreated, these deposits will eventually cause destructive changes in articular cartilage and may erode underlying bone.

Acute attacks of gout result from the deposition of uric acid crystals within a joint resulting in an acute inflammatory reaction, although the reason why this should occur from time to time remains obscure. There is a direct relationship between the severity of the hyperuricaemia and the liability to develop attacks of gout, yet many patients are found to have symptomless hyperuricaemia. Provocative factors in inducing acute gouty arthritis appear to include trauma to a joint, dietary or alcoholic excesses, surgical operations, and the intake of certain drugs.

The clinical picture is usually that of an extremely acute monarthritis, and this, together with the finding of a raised serum uric acid, is usually sufficient to make a firm diagnosis. In cases of doubt, a definitive diagnosis may be made by aspirating an affected joint (or needling a tophus), and identifying crystals of uric acid under polarised light microscopy.

Renal disease is the most frequent complication of gout, and may vary from a mild proteinuria to the deposition of urates within the kidney with vascular changes or pyelonephritis. In addition, there is some evidence of an increased liability to hypertension and arterial disease in those patients with significantly raised levels of serum uric acid.

Chondrocalcinosis (pseudo-gout, or calcium gout) is another form of crystal synovitis, less common than uric acid gout, and due to the local deposition of crystals of calcium pyrophosphate dihydrate. As in true gout, the typical crystals may be identified in joint fluid or within leucocytes. The metabolic disturbance underlying the disease is unknown, but it may be associated with uric acid gout, hypertension, diabetes mellitus, or hyperparathyroidism. In cases not associated with other conditions, biochemical studies are remarkable for their normality.

Unlike uric acid gout, males are not predominantly affected; the clinical picture of an acute inflammatory monarthritis closely resembles true gout but larger joints – usually the knees or wrists – are most commonly affected. Occasionally the condition presents as an acute polyarthritis resembling rheumatoid arthritis, or may give rise to premature and widespread degenerative arthritis. In a small proportion of cases there appears to be a hereditary factor.

The diagnosis should be suspected in any middle aged woman who develops a sudden and acute inflammatory arthritis of one or other knee joint. It can be confirmed by aspiration of the affected joint and finding the typical weakly positive birefringent crystals in the joint fluid, or by the radiological exhibition of calcification within joint menisci or articular cartilage.

Apart from chondrocalcinosis, calcification of articular cartilage may be seen in other conditions – notably following renal dialysis.

GOUT

101 Crystals of uric acid seen under polarised light microscopy.

102 Acute gout affecting the metatarsophalangeal joint of the great toe. Redness, swelling and pain are usually intense.

103 Chronic tophaceous gout Note deposits of uric acid visible beneath the skin of the fingers. From time to time these tophi may ulcerate through the skin and exude a white chalky material, in which urate crystals can be identified.

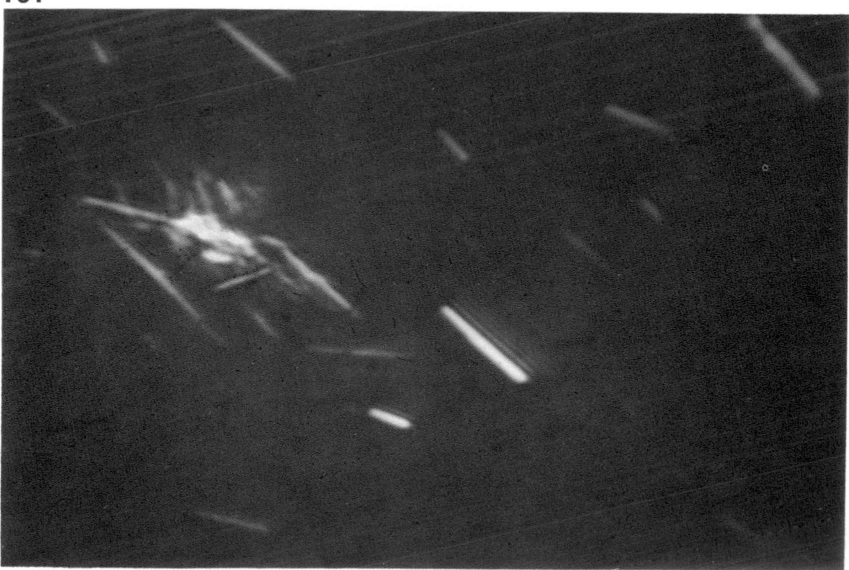

102

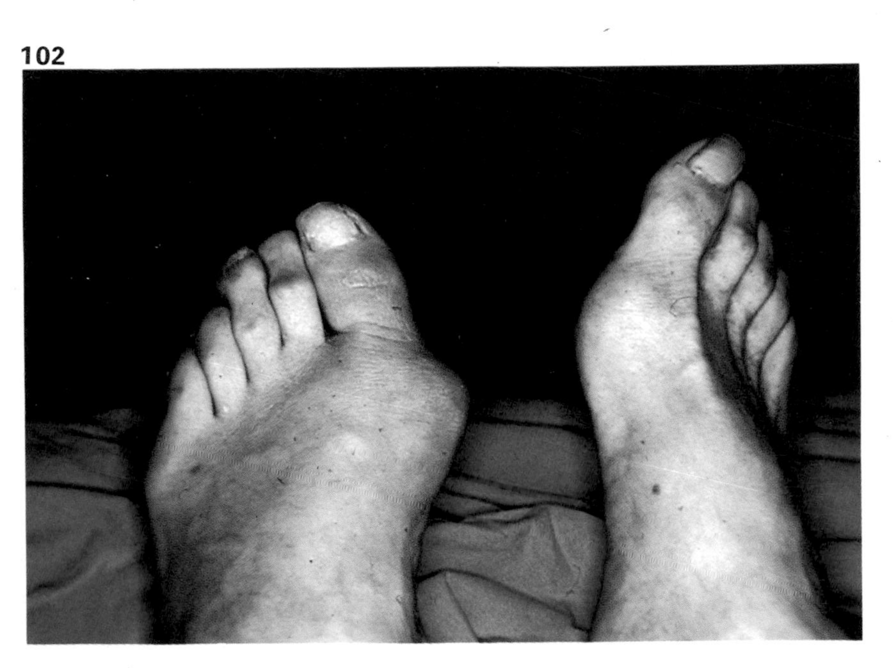

103

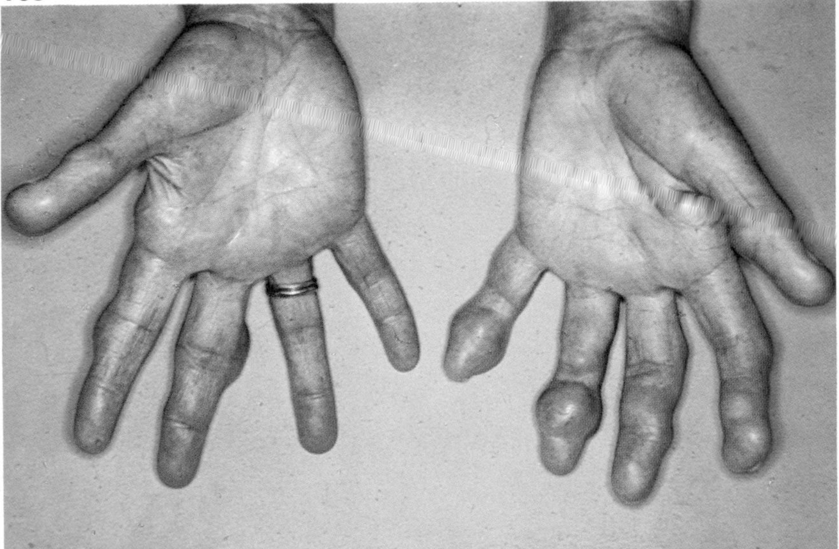

104 X-ray of the right hand in the previous illustration. Deposits of uric acid are just visible in the soft tissues, and 'punched out' areas in adjacent bone are seen.

105 Similar tophaceous deposits around chronic gouty halluces.

106 Tophaceous deposits on the ear Deposits may appear in cartilage away from joints, in the tarsal plate of the eye, or in the nasal cartilage.

107 Enlargement of the olecranon bursae may also be a feature of chronic gout, and tophaceous deposits may be demonstrated therein.

104

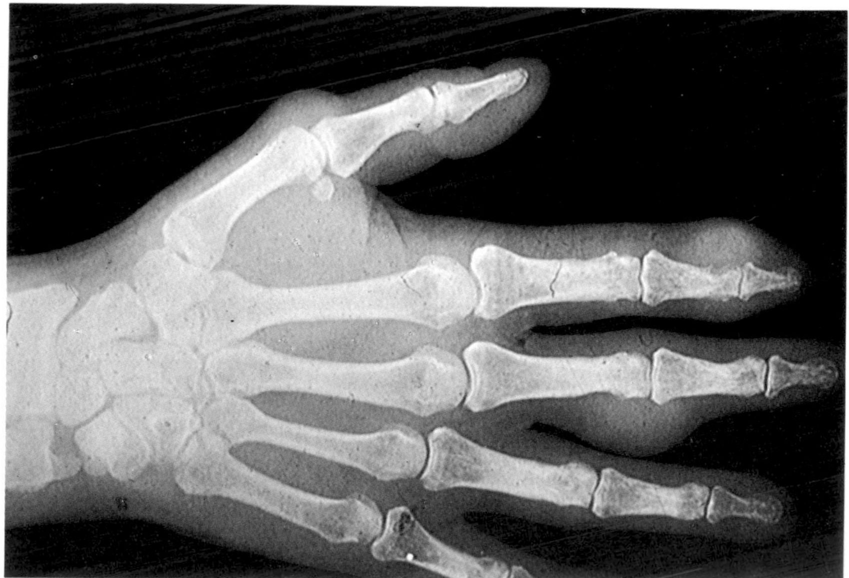

105

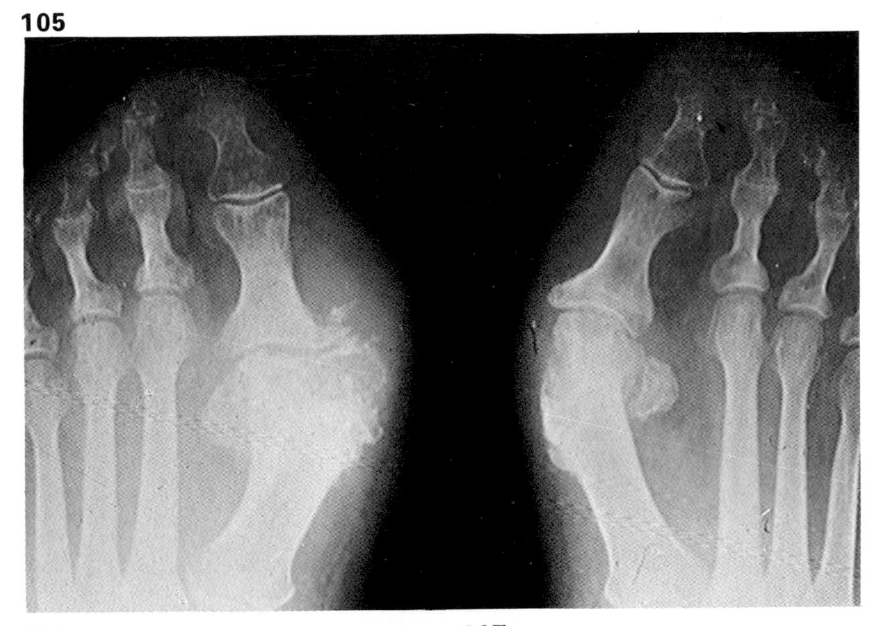

106

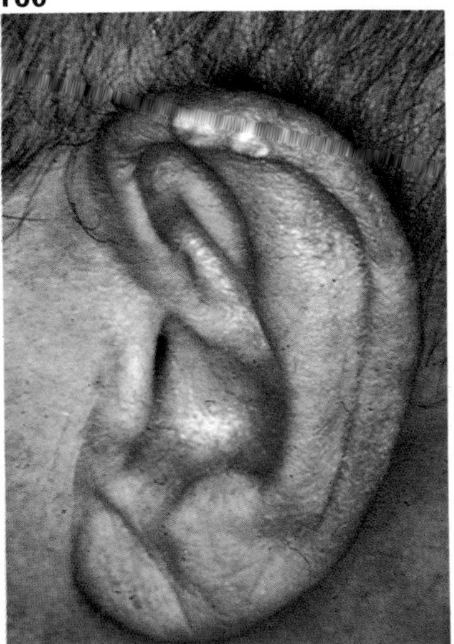

107

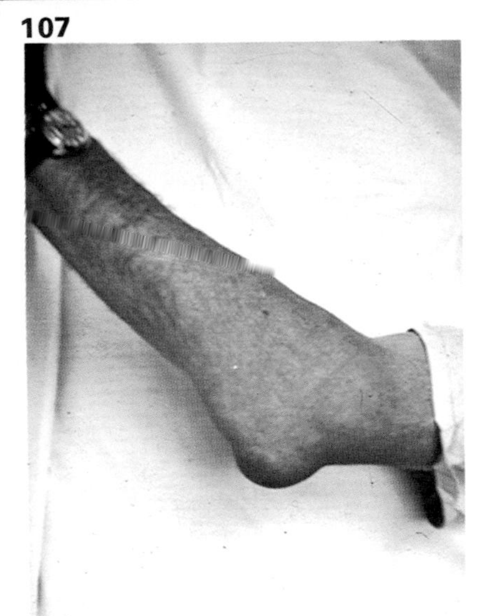

CHONDROCALCINOSIS

108 Characteristic x-ray appearance of the knee joint in chondrocalcinosis Calcification is seen in both menisci in the antero-posterior view, while in the lateral view a thin rim of calcification is seen in the articular cartilage on the posterior aspect of the femoral condyle.

109 Enlarged view of the above shows the calcification in the articular cartilage of the femoral condyle.

110 The wrist in chondrocalcinosis Calcification is seen in the triangular ligament.

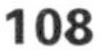

108

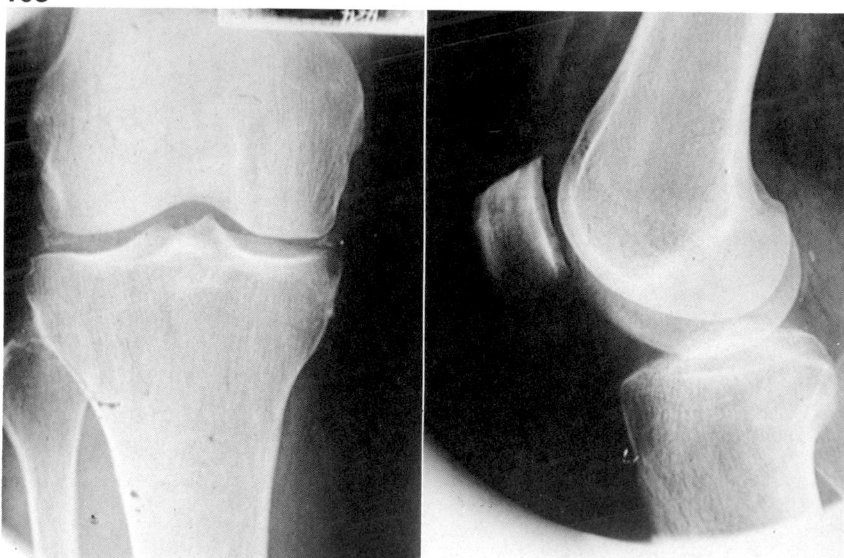

109

110

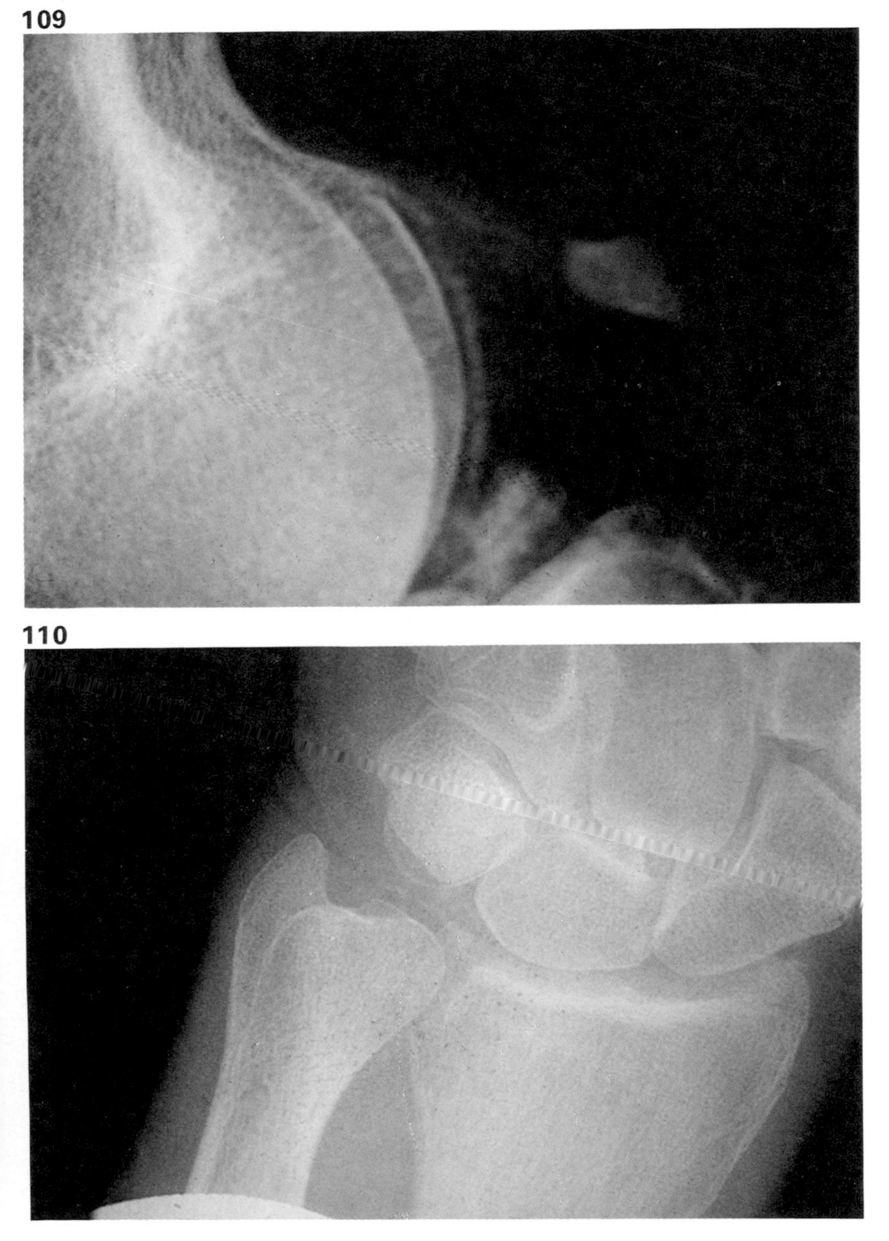

111 A rhomboidal crystal of calcium pyrophosphate dihydrate ingested by a leucocyte, seen in the aspirate from an affected joint under polarised light microscopy.

111

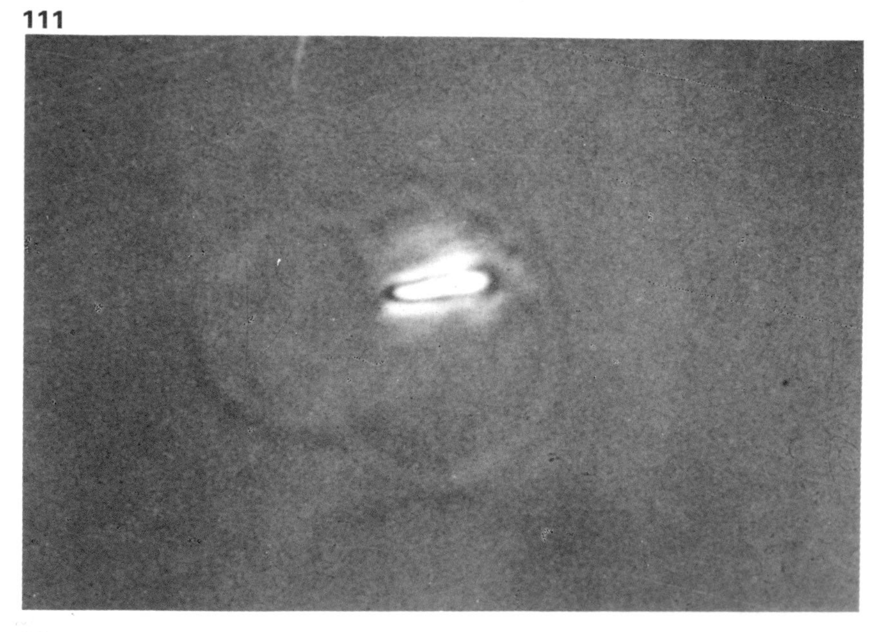

Connective Tissue Disorders

In the following chapter are illustrated four of the more important connective tissue disorders – systemic lupus erythematosus, systemic sclerosis, polyarteritis nodosa, and polymyositis or dermatomyositis.

Connective tissue is composed essentially of collagen, elastic fibres and fibroblasts in an amorphous ground substance. A common thread is seen to run through the histological changes in these diseases, particularly the widespread vascular pathology and the fibrinoid change in the ground substance. Consequently they have many clinical features in common, and it is not always possible to decide with certainty into which diagnostic category a patient may fall.

With the exception of progressive systemic sclerosis the advent of steroid therapy has vastly improved the prognosis of these diseases which previously resulted so often in a fatal outcome.

Each is a multi-system disease with a widely variable clinical picture, but the major features of each (there are many others), may be summarised as follows:

Systemic lupus erythematosus : fever, arthralgia or arthritis, skin rashes, proteinuria, polyserositis, hepato-splenomegaly, and psychiatric disturbances.

Progressive systemic sclerosis : thickening of the skin and telangiectasia, Raynaud's phenomenon, dysphagia, subcutaneous calcinosis, and renal failure.

Polyarteritis nodosa : fever, muscle and joint pains, bronchial asthma, abdominal pain, hypertension, renal disease, and mononeuritis multiplex.

Polymyositis or dermatomyositis : profound proximal muscle weakness, muscle pain and tenderness, arthralgia or arthritis, dusky erythema of the face, upper arms and thorax, and violaceous discoloration around nail beds.

The illustrations which follow show some of the more important clinical and histological features of these diseases.

SYSTEMIC LUPUS ERYTHEMATOSUS

S.L.E. is a multi-system disease which may present in a variety of ways. The most constant features are fever, arthralgia or arthritis, skin rashes, and polyserositis. There is no constant pattern of the disease and diagnosis may be difficult.

The pattern of joint symptoms and signs is variable, sometimes presenting as a flitting mono-or polyarthritis, and sometimes being clinically indistinguishable from rheumatoid arthritis. Often the degree of pain complained of by the patient is much more than would be expected from the physician's examination – a feature which should lead one to suspect the disease.

The butterfly rash on the face is the most typical skin manifestation, but non-specific or petechial rashes may also occur on other parts of the body. Alopecia, localised or generalised, may occur.

Episodes of chest pain, in the absence of either clinical or radiological signs, may occur. Pleural and pericardial effusions signify a polyserositis, and myocarditis or aortic insufficiency may lead to cardiac failure.

Psychoses or actual fits may occur, but peripheral neuropathies are less common than in rheumatoid arthritis.

The most serious feature of the disease is renal involvement, usually heralded by the advent of proteinuria, and if progressive, it may determine a fatal outcome. It is found in about 75% of cases coming to autopsy.

112 The L.E. cell (seen here) is only found in 75% of cases, and a more reliable test is the anti-nuclear antibody which is positive in about 95% of cases. Other important indicators of the disease are a very high E.S.R., leucopenia and false positive W.R.

113 The 'butterfly rash' is the most common skin manifestation of S.L.E. This is a sunlight sensitive rash occurring over the bridge of the nose and the cheeks. Note the bulbous eruption around the lips.

114 The forearms and other areas exposed to sunlight may be affected.

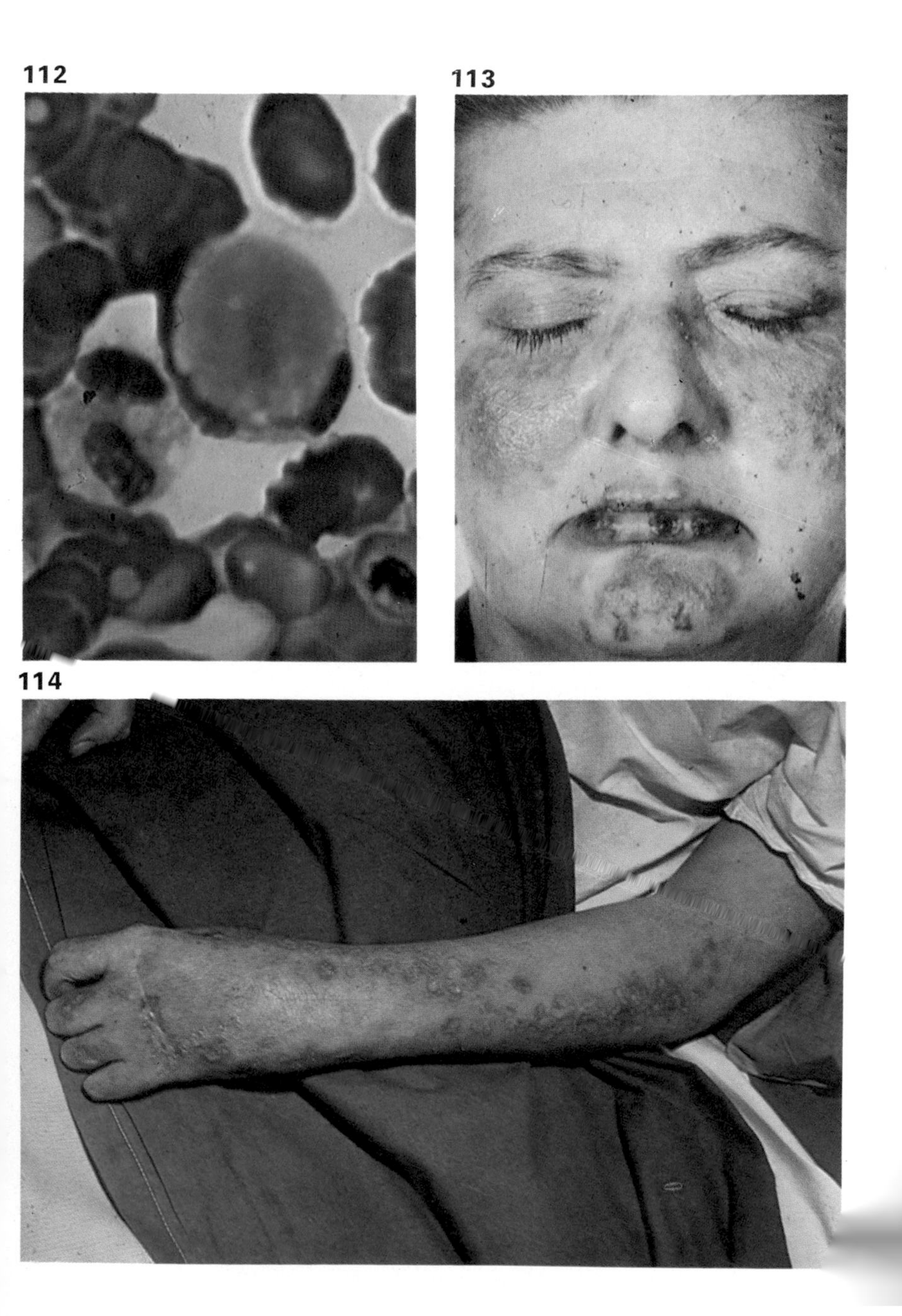
112
113
114

115 The hands of a patient with proven S.L.E. There was severe pain in the small joints of the hands for two years, yet apart from minor cartilage loss no destructive changes are apparent. The arthritis of S.L.E. may take several forms. It sometimes closely resembles the polyarthritis of rheumatoid disease, but may be transient and flitting as in rheumatic fever, or simply present as a severe arthralgia without supporting signs of inflammation. Radiologically, the affected joints show surprisingly little change. cartilage loss and erosions often being long delayed or absent.

116 The 'wire loop' lesion Focal glomerulitis is followed by an increase in the thickness of the basement membrane and tubular degeneration. The final picture is that of chronic glomerulonephritis. Many patients develop a protein-losing kidney of the nephrotic syndrome type, while others may have a pyelonephritis which may be mistaken for S.L.E. nephritis.

115

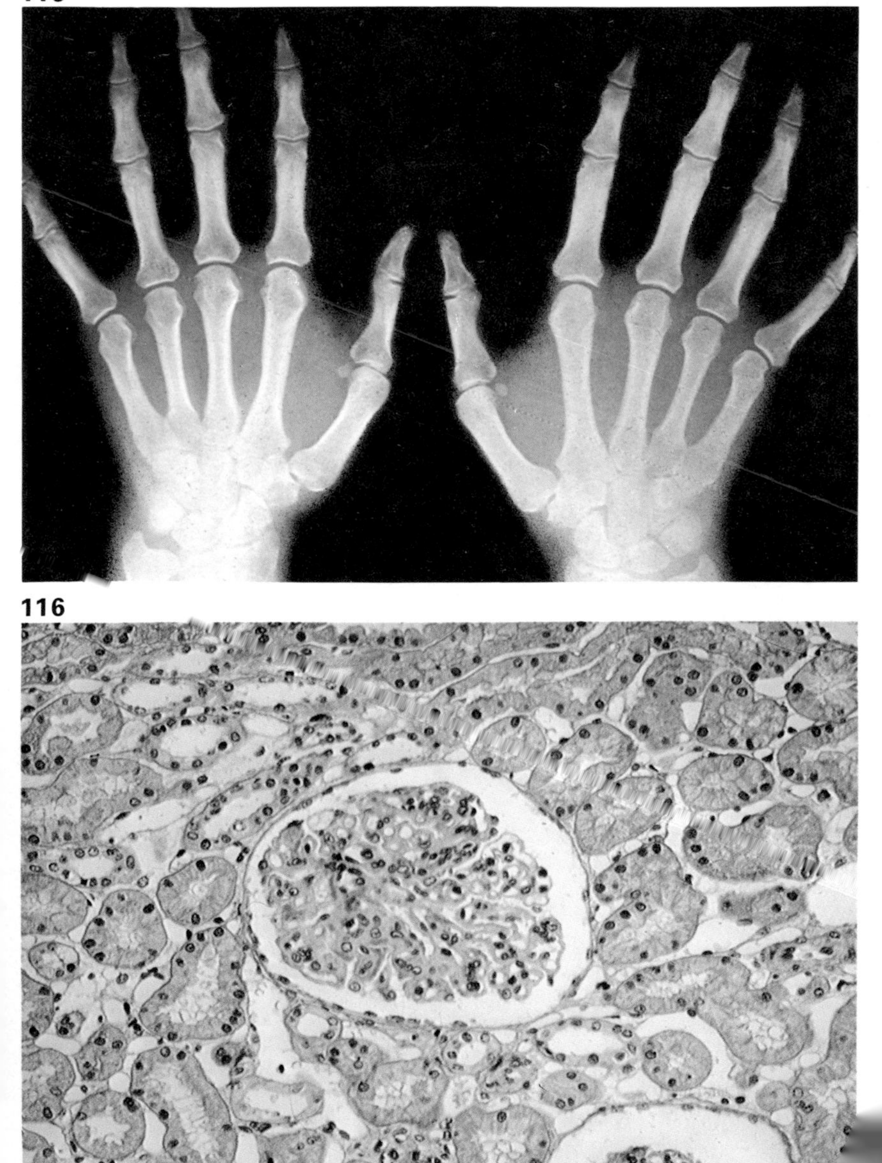

116

PROGRESSIVE SYSTEMIC SCLEROSIS (SCLERODERMA)

The characteristic features of this disease are thickening of the skin of the extremities, Raynaud's phenomenon, subcutaneous calcific deposits, and telangiectasis. Like S.L.E., it may progress to a multi-system disease with pulmonary, cardiac, and gastro-intestinal manifestations. Polymyositis and peripheral neuropathies may complicate the picture, and present an apparent overlap with other connective tissue disorders.

117 Early scleroderma of the fingers The skin is thickened, waxy in appearance, and bound down to underlying tissue.

118 Advanced scleroderma of the hands Necrosis of terminal phalanges has occurred from ischaemia due to Raynaud's phenomenon, and the hardened skin has given rise to fixed flexion contractures.

119 Another view of the same hands Note the white deposits of calcific material under the skin indicating calcinosis.

117

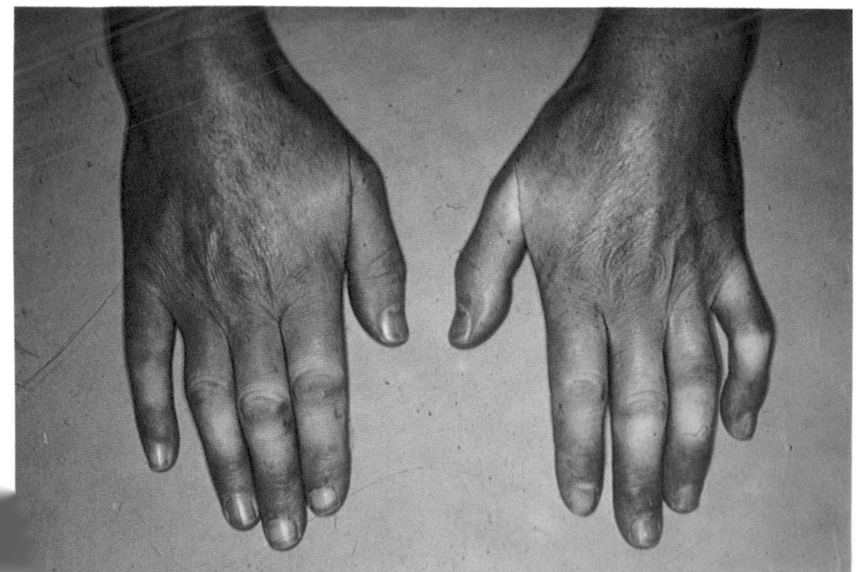

118

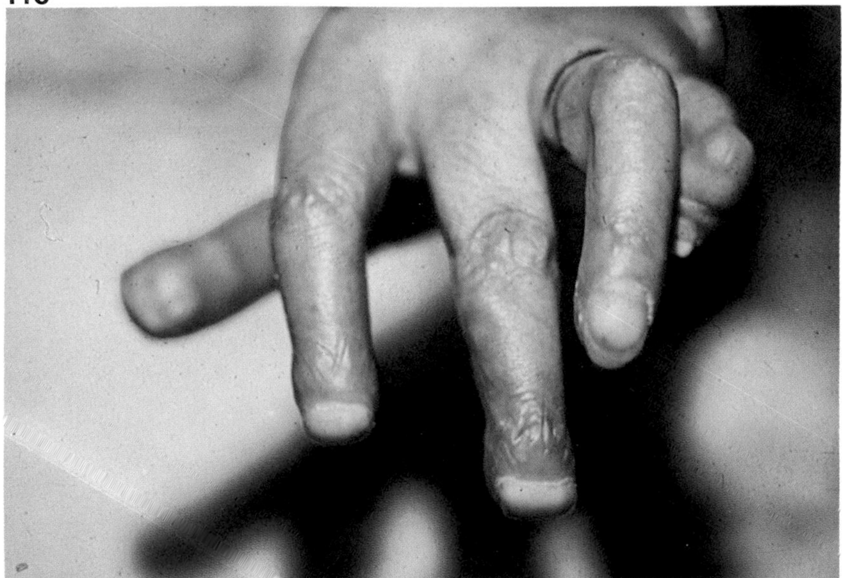

119

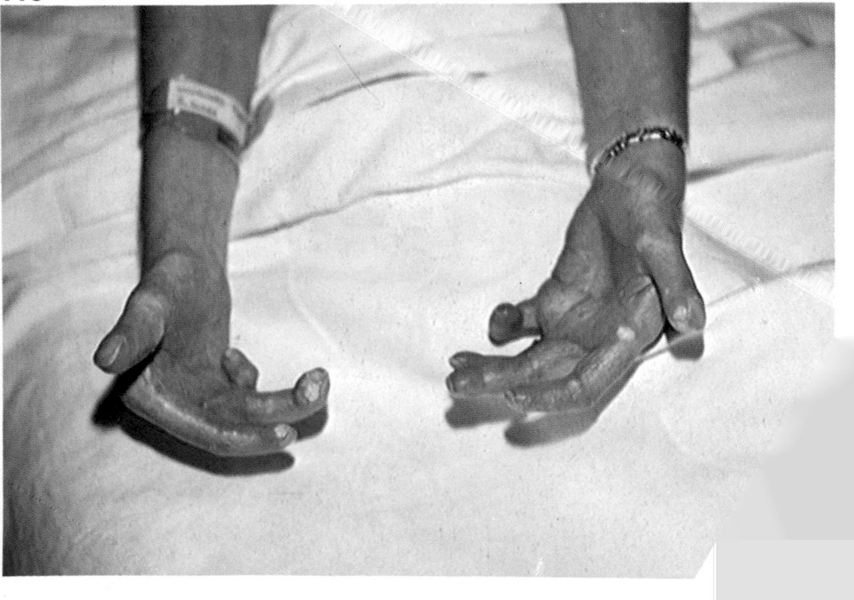

120 The face in advanced scleroderma shows induration of the skin and telangiectasia on the cheeks and nose.

121 Dysphagia is common due to involvement of the oesophagus in the fibrotic process. Barium swallow x-ray shows narrowing and lack of peristalsis.

122 The hands in scleroderma There is (1) necrosis of the terminal phalanx of the right index finger; and (2) early calcific deposits in the pulps of both thumbs.

123 Advanced scleroderma shows necrosis of several terminal phalanges, flexion contractures, and widespread, heavy calcific deposits.

120

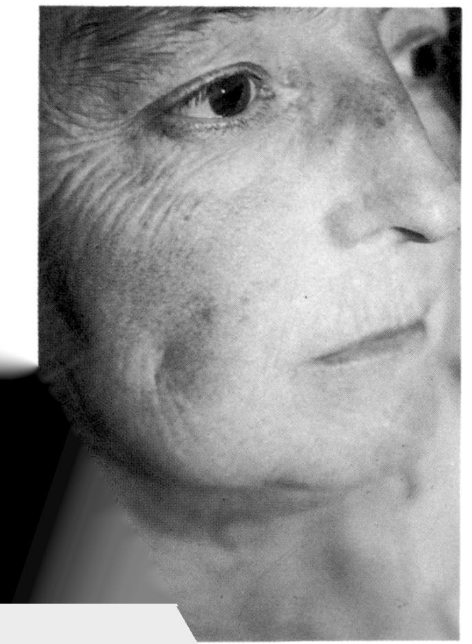

121

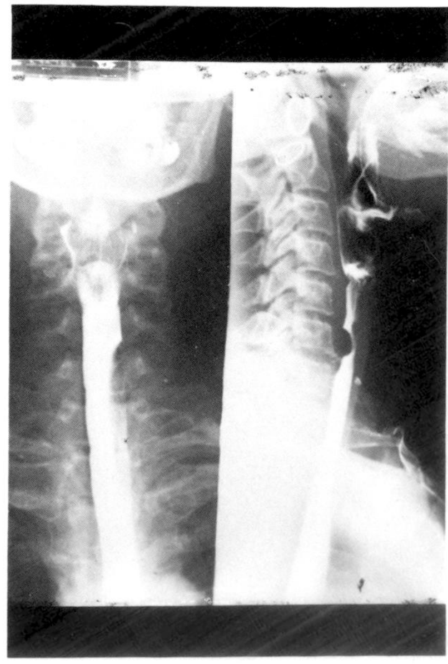

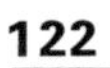

122

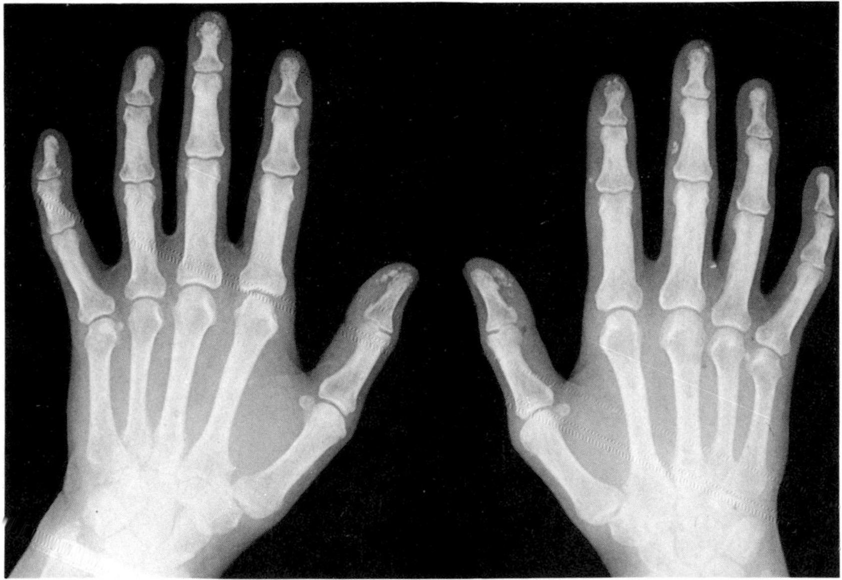

123

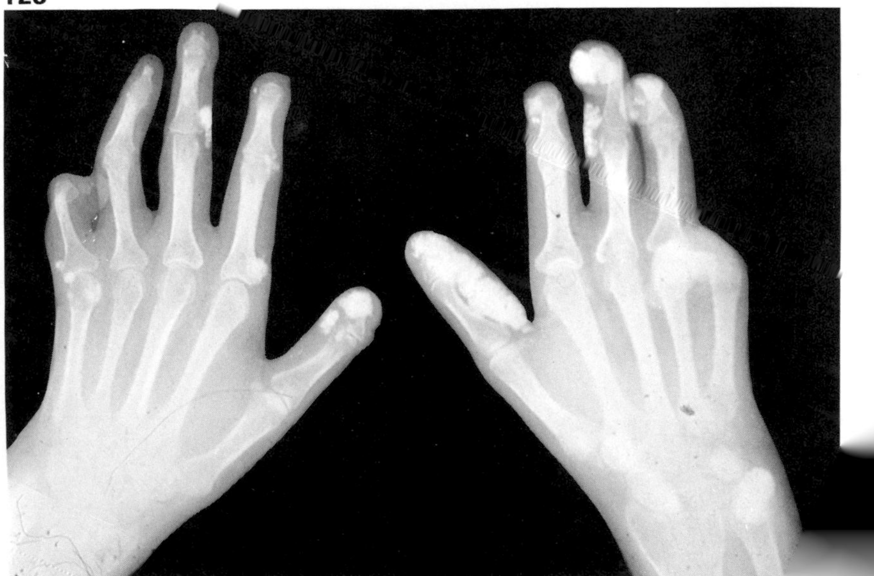

124 Section of kidney in progressive systemic sclerosis The typical renal lesion is heralded by the onset of a malignant hypertension, rapidly followed by proteinuria and a rising blood urea. The outstanding lesion on microscopical examination is intimal hyperplasia with fibrinoid necrosis of the small arteries leading to occlusion (seen in upper right of illustration). These changes are identical with those found in malignant nephrosclerosis and carry the same serious prognosis.

125 Section of skin in scleroderma Note loss of rete pegs and dense thickening of dermal collagen, with loss of adnexal structures. Note also that fibrosis extends below the level of the sweat gland seen lower left centre.

124

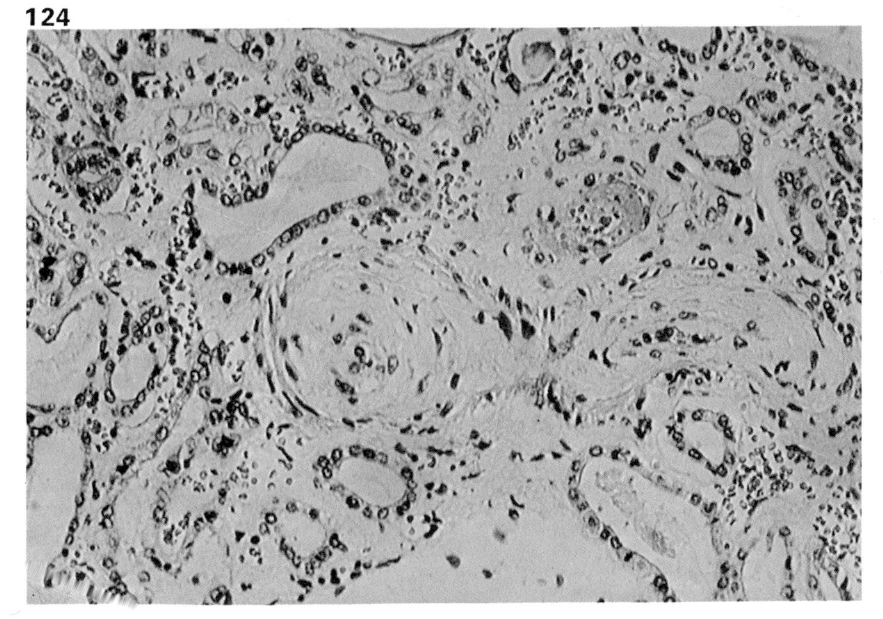

125

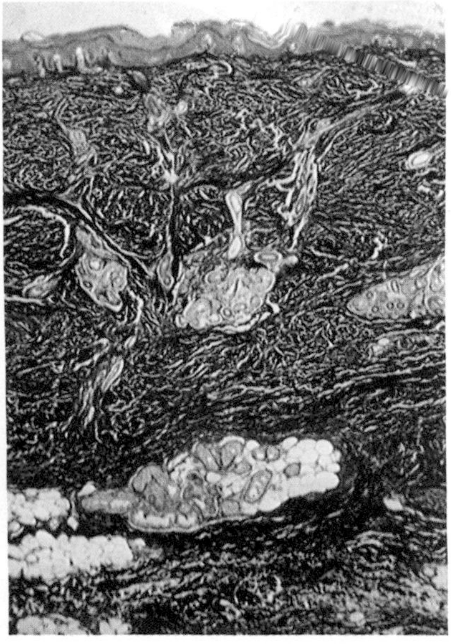

POLYARTERITIS NODOSA

Of all the connective tissue disorders, this in particular has been looked upon as a hypersensitivity disease. The initial symptoms are so diverse that diagnosis is usually difficult. Unexplained fever, hypertension, muscle and joint pains, asthma, peripheral neuropathies, or acute abdominal pain may each be the presenting feature. Renal involvement is a later phenomenon.

The basic pathology involves the small and medium sized arteries with inflammatory changes in the media, later involving both the intima and adventitia. Destruction of the internal elastic lamina may follow, giving rise to thrombosis, or weakening of the arterial wall and aneurysm formation.

Possible related forms of primary arterial disease include cranial arteritis, Takayasu's disease (aortic arch syndrome), and Wegener's granulomatosis.

126 Typical changes of inflammation of all coats of the vessel. Note destruction of the internal elastic lamina and proliferation of the intima. This often proceeds to thrombosis in the vessel.

127 Focal glomerulo-nephritis with marked distortion of the structure of the tuft. As in the previous two diseases, renal involvement is common, occurring in over 60% of patients. Proteinuria and/or haematuria may precede hypertension and lead to renal failure.

128 Another section of kidney shows a renal inter-lobular artery with necrosis and heavy cellular infiltration of the wall.

129 Temporal arteritis (cranial arteritis) Biopsy of a temporal artery shows diffuse fibrosis of the intima with narrowing of the lumen of the vessel. The media shows inflammatory changes proceeding to focal necrosis, and giant cells may be present. This may be a benign variant of polyarteritis, occurring in an older age group. Apart from unilateral or bilateral severe temporal headache, there is often a systemic disturbance with malaise, weight loss, muscle pain and fever.

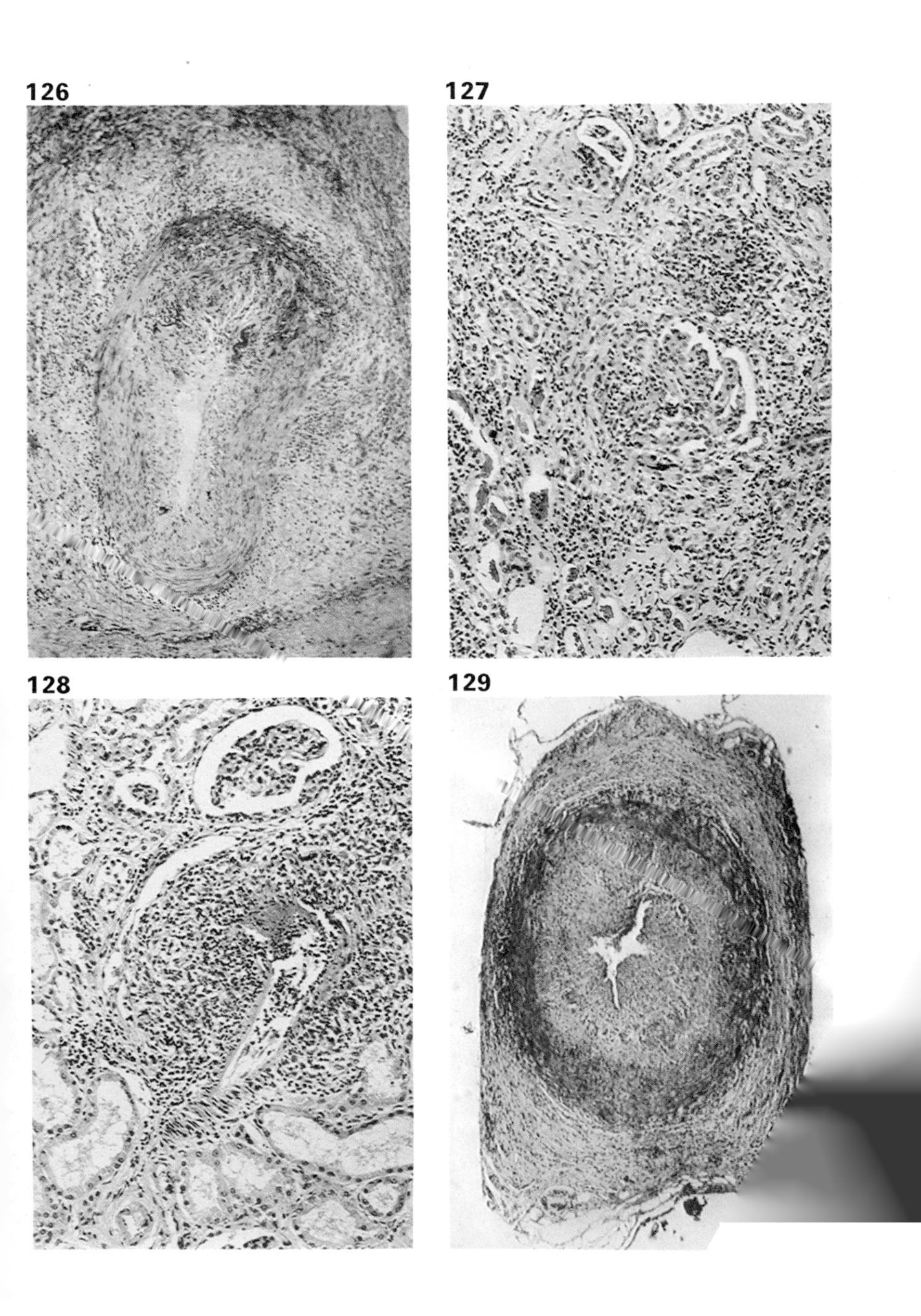
126
127
128
129

POLYMYOSITIS

In polymyositis, the primary pathology is an inflammatory and degenerative change in skeletal muscles. The outstanding clinical feature is pain in the proximal limb segments, and examination discloses tenderness and usually profound weakness of the limbs. Polymyositis may appear as an apparently primary condition, but may also be found as part of other connective tissue disorders, especially scleroderma. Dermatomyositis is a closely related disease, in which, in addition to the findings in the muscles, an oedematous dusky red erythema occurs affecting the face and upper trunk. Both conditions, especially dermatomyositis, have a known association with malignant disease, and may precede the appearance of the latter by many months. Apart from alteration in muscle enzymes, the diagnosis may be established by muscle biopsy.

130 Typical changes of fragmented and degenerate muscle fibres lie in a background of fibrous tissue heavily infiltrated by leucocytes.

131 The hands in dermatomyositis Patchy erythema on the dorsum of the digits, with violaceous discoloration of the nail beds is typical.

132 The facial eruption of dermatomyositis The rash is a dusky erythema involving particularly the peri-orbital region and forehead, but may also occur in the neck, shoulders or arms.

130

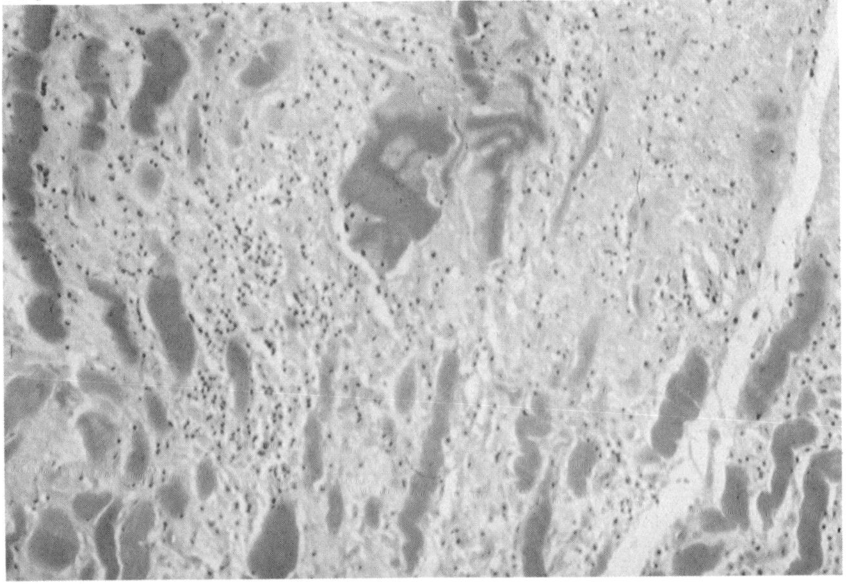

131

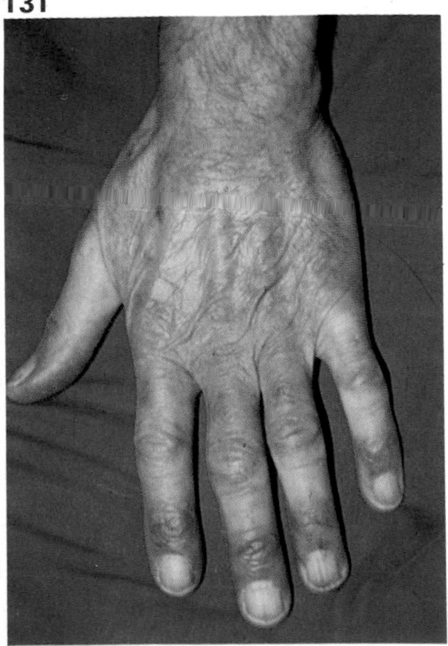

132

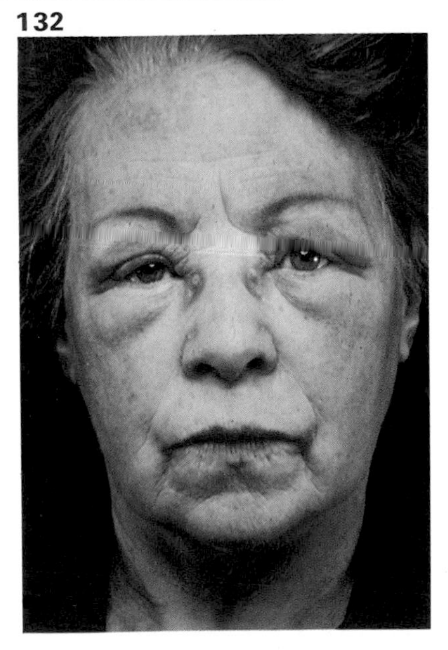

133 Close-up of the same patient showing the typical heliotrope discoloration and oedema of the peri-orbital region.

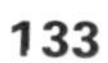

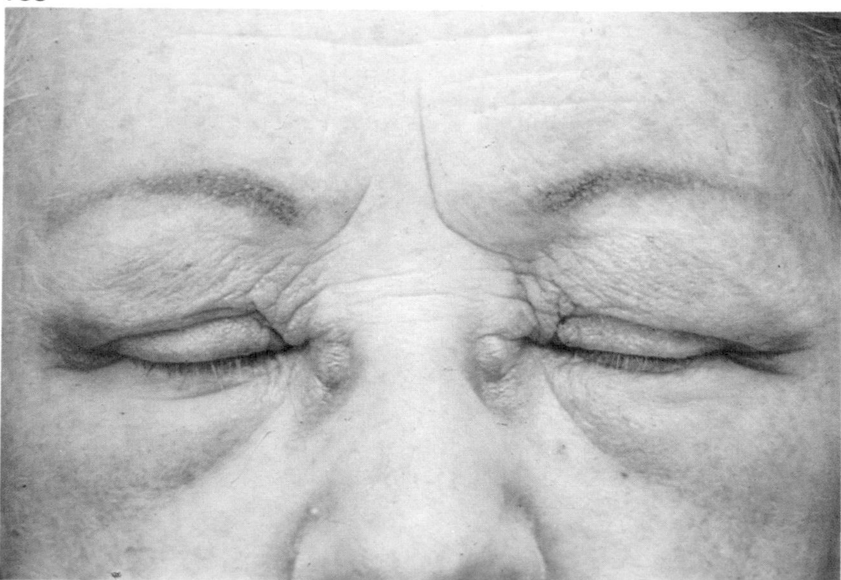

Rarer forms of Arthritis

There are more than 100 diseases with which an arthritis may be associated, and the list on page 9 shows the more important of these. Thus an inflammatory arthritis may complicate viral infections such as rubella or glandular fever, bacterial infections as in brucellosis, gonorrhoea, or the salmonella group, hypersensitivity states, or the connective tissue disorders.

An arthritis of degenerative type may occur in endocrine disorders – e.g. acromegaly, or in various metabolic diseases such as haemochromatosis. The list is large, and an underlying primary disease must always be considered if an arthritis appears in any way to vary from the common pattern.

The chapter which follows describes a few diseases in which affection of joints is by no means uncommon, and which may trap the unwary clinician.

ACROMEGALIC ARTHRITIS

Joint pain and muscle weakness are common features of this condition.

134 Large spade-like hands There is widening of joint spaces due to hypertrophy of cartilage, tufting of terminal phalanges, and spicule osteophytes at joint margins together with ossification at muscle attachments.

HYPERTROPHIC PULMONARY OSTEOARTHROPATHY

Although occasionally an hereditary condition, this is usually associated with intra-thoracic disease, commonly bronchial carcinoma or cyanotic heart disease, but may also occur in chronic bowel disease.

135 A fine periosteal frill along the sides of the phalanges is the characteristic appearance on x-ray. Clubbing of the finger nails proceeds to tenderness and thickening of the digits. These changes sometimes spread to involve the lower ends of the radius and ulna.

134

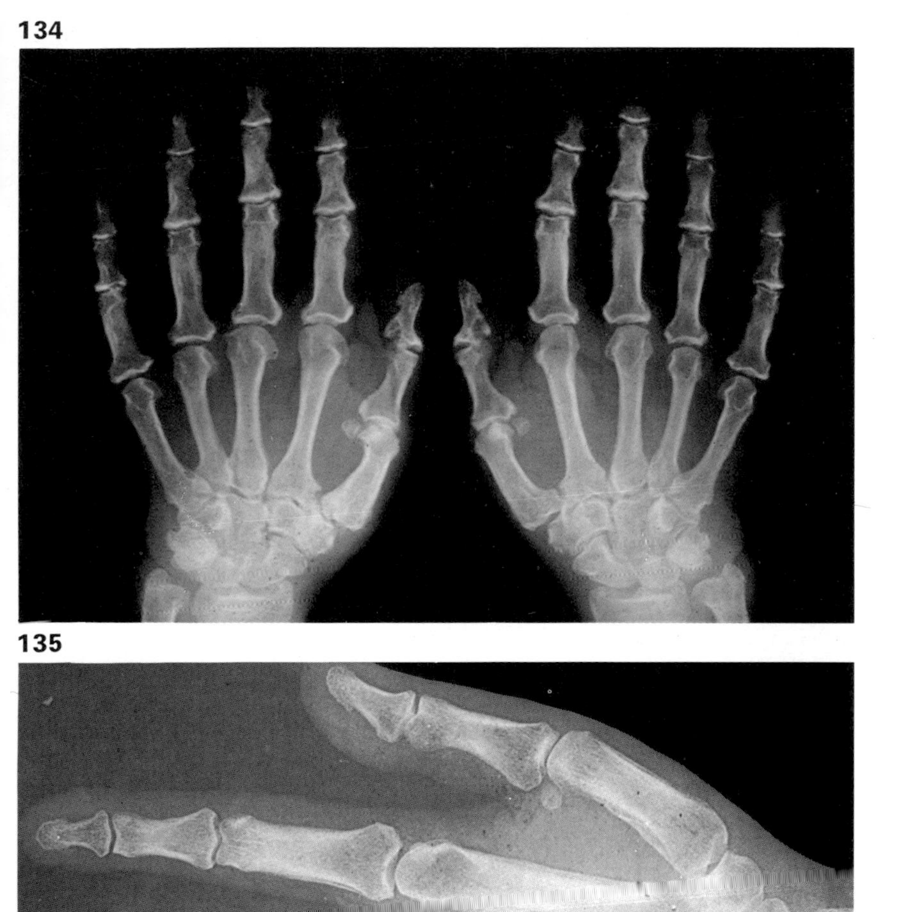

135

NEUROPATHIC ARTHRITIS

Syphilis, diabetes and syringomyelia are the most common causes of neuropathic arthritis. In syphilis, the large weight bearing joints—lumbar spine, hips and knees—are most commonly affected ; in diabetes, the small joints of the foot ; and in syringomyelia, the joints of the upper limb. Less common causes include peroneal muscular atrophy and various peripheral neuropathies.

136 Patient with tabes dorsalis shows early changes of destruction and fragmentation affecting the lateral tibial condyle.

137 Same patient in a more advanced stage Fragmentation now affects the tibial plateau.

138 Tabetic neuropathic arthritis of both hips Gross destructive changes, together with massive formation of new bone in bizarre pattern around the joints.

136

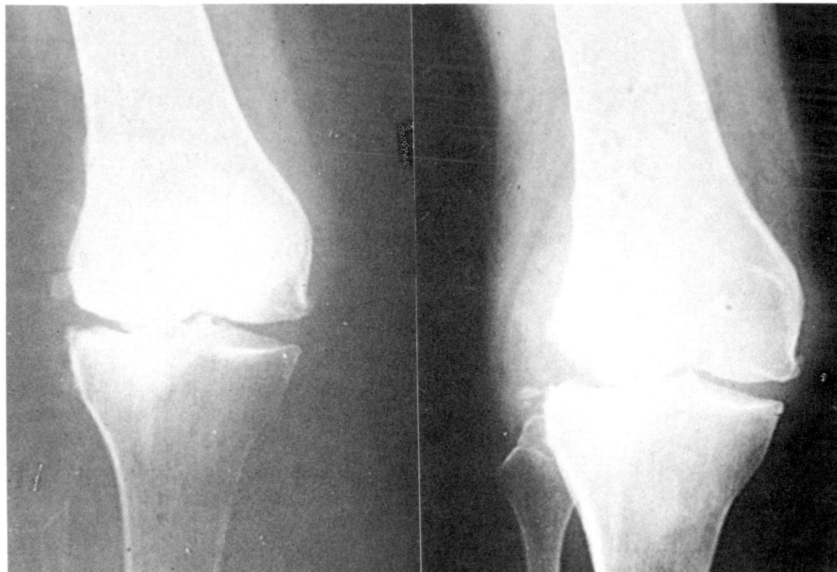

137

138

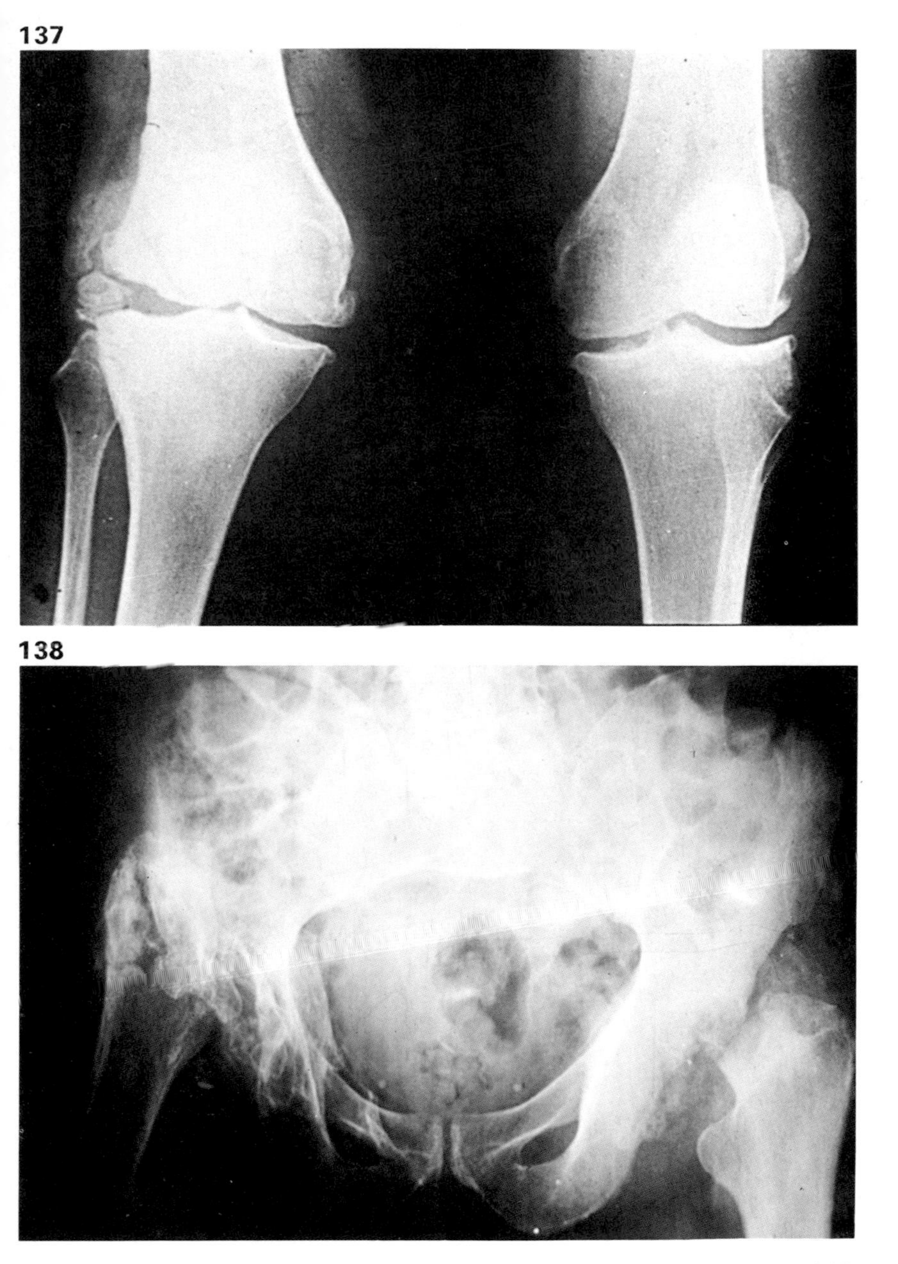

139 Neuropathic arthritis of the elbow in syringomyelia The joint was clinically disorganised but painless on movement.

140 X-ray of the above elbow Destructive changes, gross new bone formation, and disorganisation of the joint are apparent.

141 Neuropathic arthritis of the ankle joint Again destructive changes with exuberant new bone formation are seen.

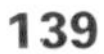

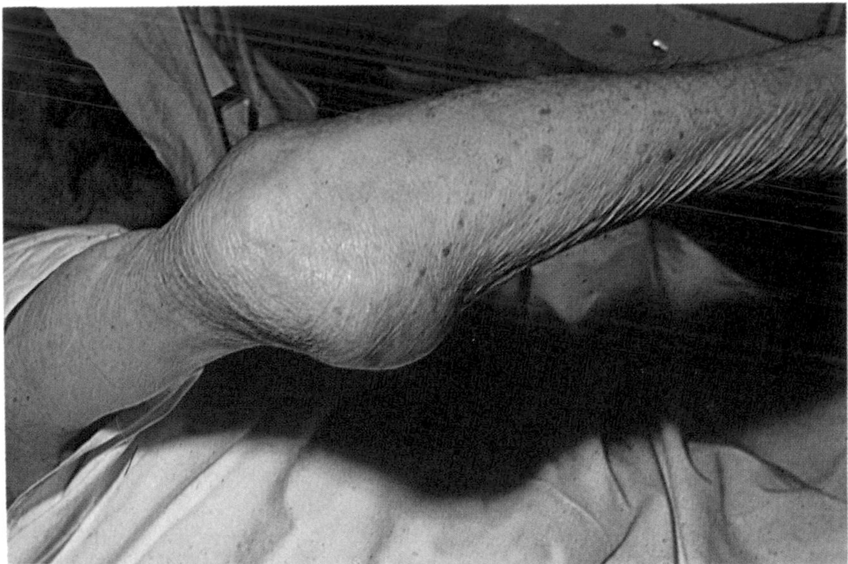

140

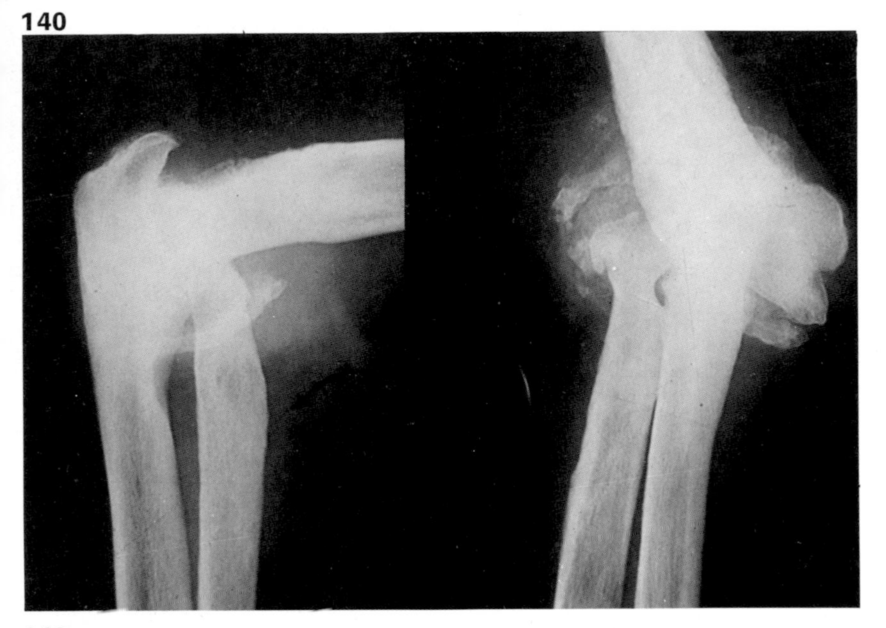

141

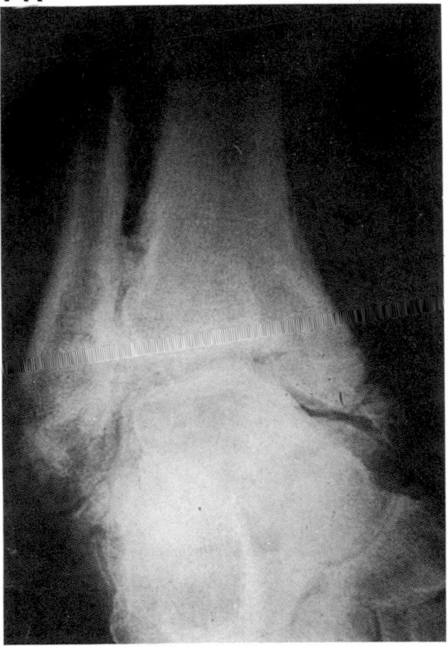

SARCOIDOSIS

Apart from its other manifestations such as malaise, cough, chest pain or erythema nodosum, sarcoidosis may affect muscles, bones or joints. Symptoms from muscle involvement usually amount to no more than vague aches and pains, but proximal myopathy has been described. Sarcoid of bone is usually symptomless. Arthropathy most commonly involves the knees and ankles, presenting as a symmetrical periarthritis or synovitis, and often precedes the onset of erythema nodosum.

Joint manifestations most commonly affect the spinal column, giving the appearance of severe spondylosis. Kyphosis and ultimate rigidity of the spine results from calcification and, finally, ossification of the intervertebral discs.

Severe degenerative changes in the peripheral joints may also occur, involving the knees, hips, and shoulders.

142 Central punched out areas in the phalanges are the most typical radiological change.

143 Fine lacework bone pattern in the phalanges, seen here in the middle phalanx of the ring finger, is another radiological feature in sarcoidosis.

This term describes the pigmentation of cartilage which occurs in those who suffer from alkaptonuria. Clinical symptoms and signs usually develop in early middle life. Bluish-black discoloration may affect the cartilage of the ears, nasal cartilage, the hard palate or the sclerae.

144 Pigmentation of the nose is apparent

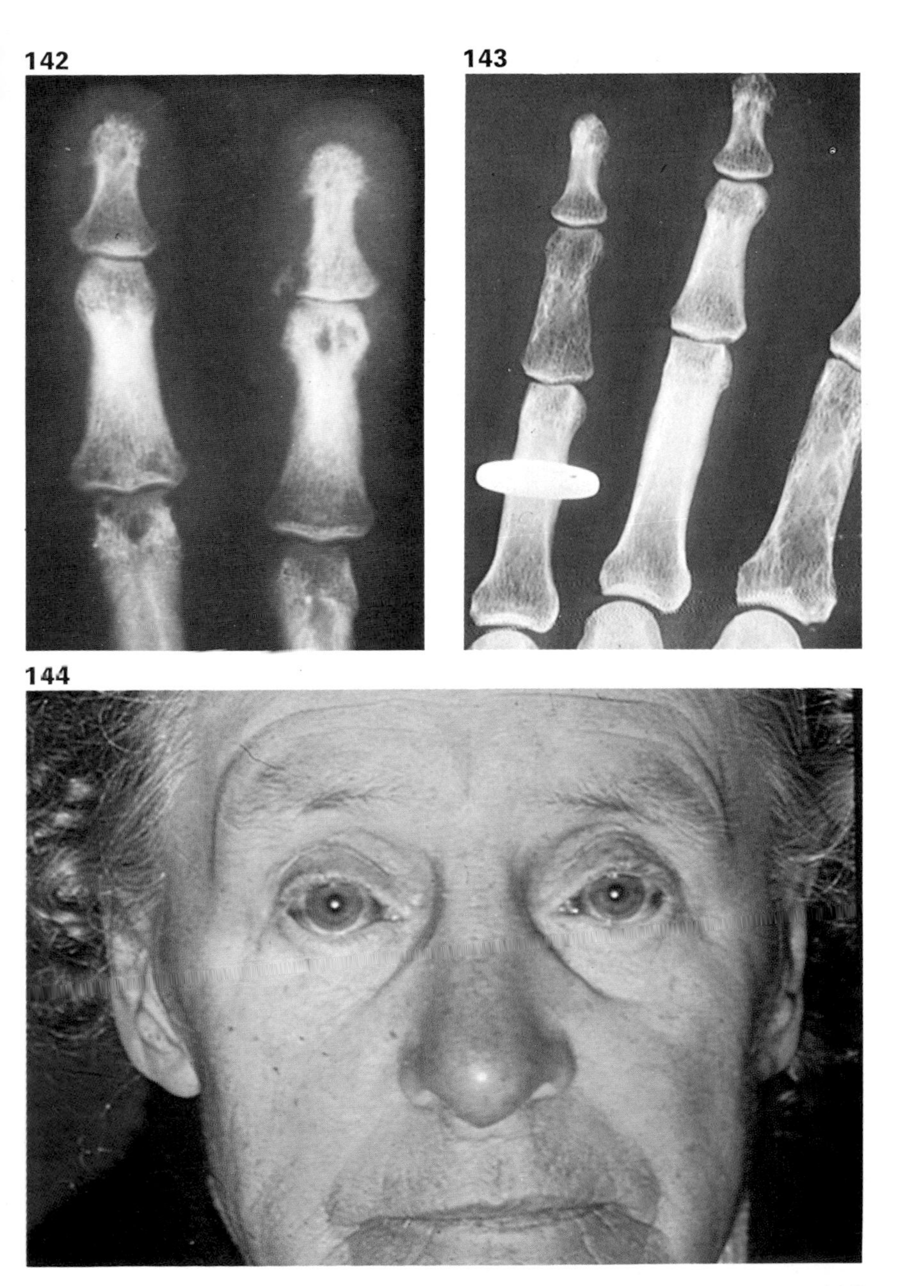
142
143
144

145 Close-up of the same patient shows pigmentation of the sclerae.

146 The ears of the same patient display the typical bluish-black discoloration.

147 Marked collapse and calcification of intervertebral discs Joints in ochronosis show premature and severe degenerative changes.

145

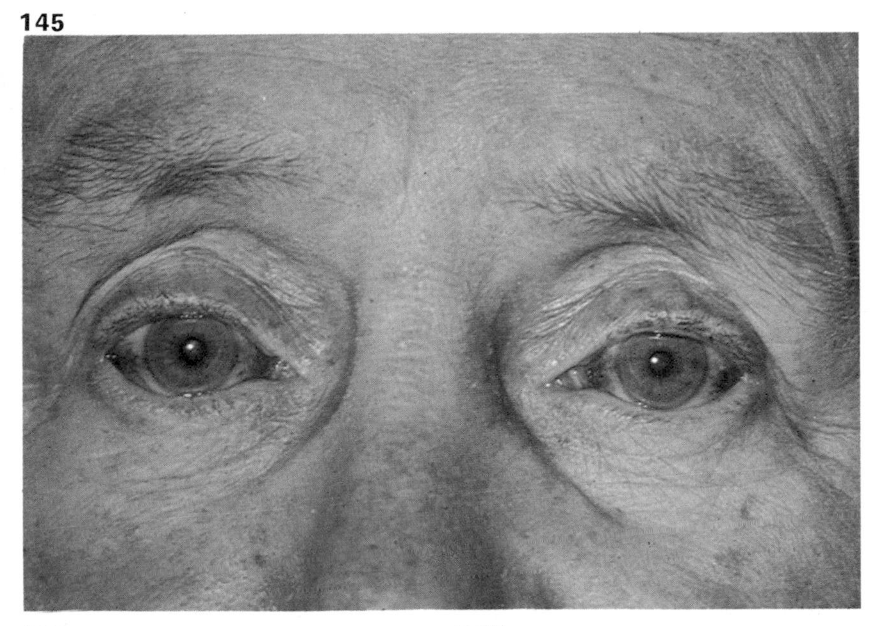

146

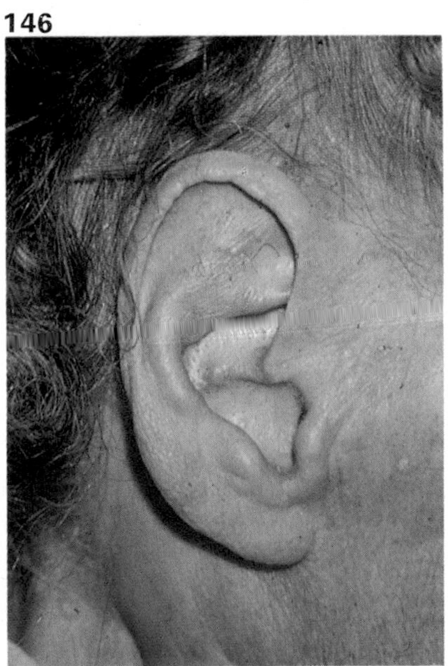

147

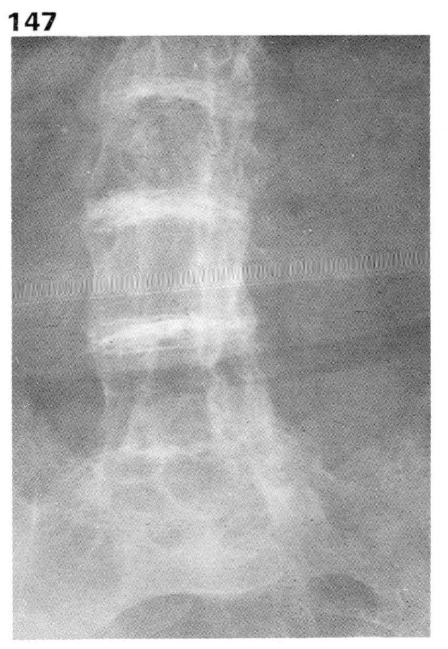

MYELOMATOSIS

Apart from bone pain in the spine and ribs, myelomatosis is occasionally accompanied by a polyarthritis with some resemblance to rheumatoid arthritis, and involving the small joints of the hands.

148 Deposits of amyloid material cause swelling of joints. Radiologically, one may see destructive changes in bone adjacent to affected joints.

HAEMOCHROMATOSIS

This disease may be associated with chondrocalcinosis (see page 90), or with a more chronic and destructive arthropathy.

149 Bone sclerosis, irregularity of the joint margins and cyst formation are seen.

148

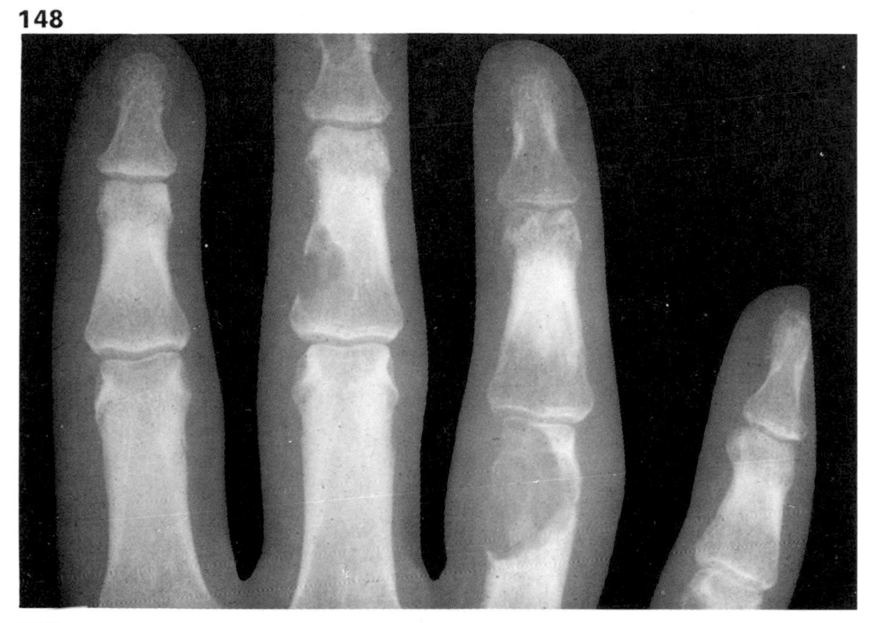

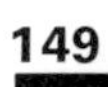

149

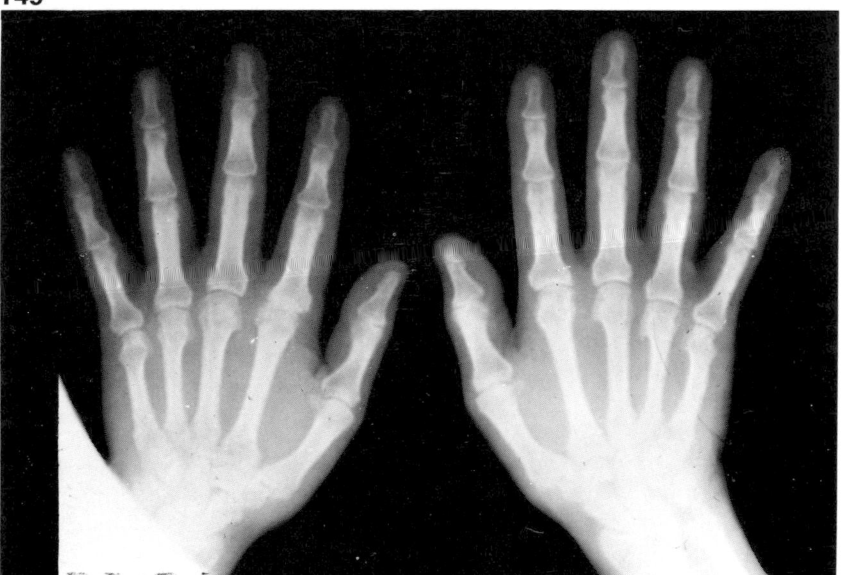

HAEMOPHILIA

The arthropathy of haemophilia is due to repeated haemarthroses. The knees, ankles, elbows, and shoulders are most commonly affected.

150 Haemophiliac knee joint Note loss of joint space, widening of the femoral inter-condylar notch and irregular sclerotic and destructive changes affecting the tibial plateau and adjacent femoral condyle.

151 The elbow in haemophilia Similar changes are seen as in the knee joint.

150

151

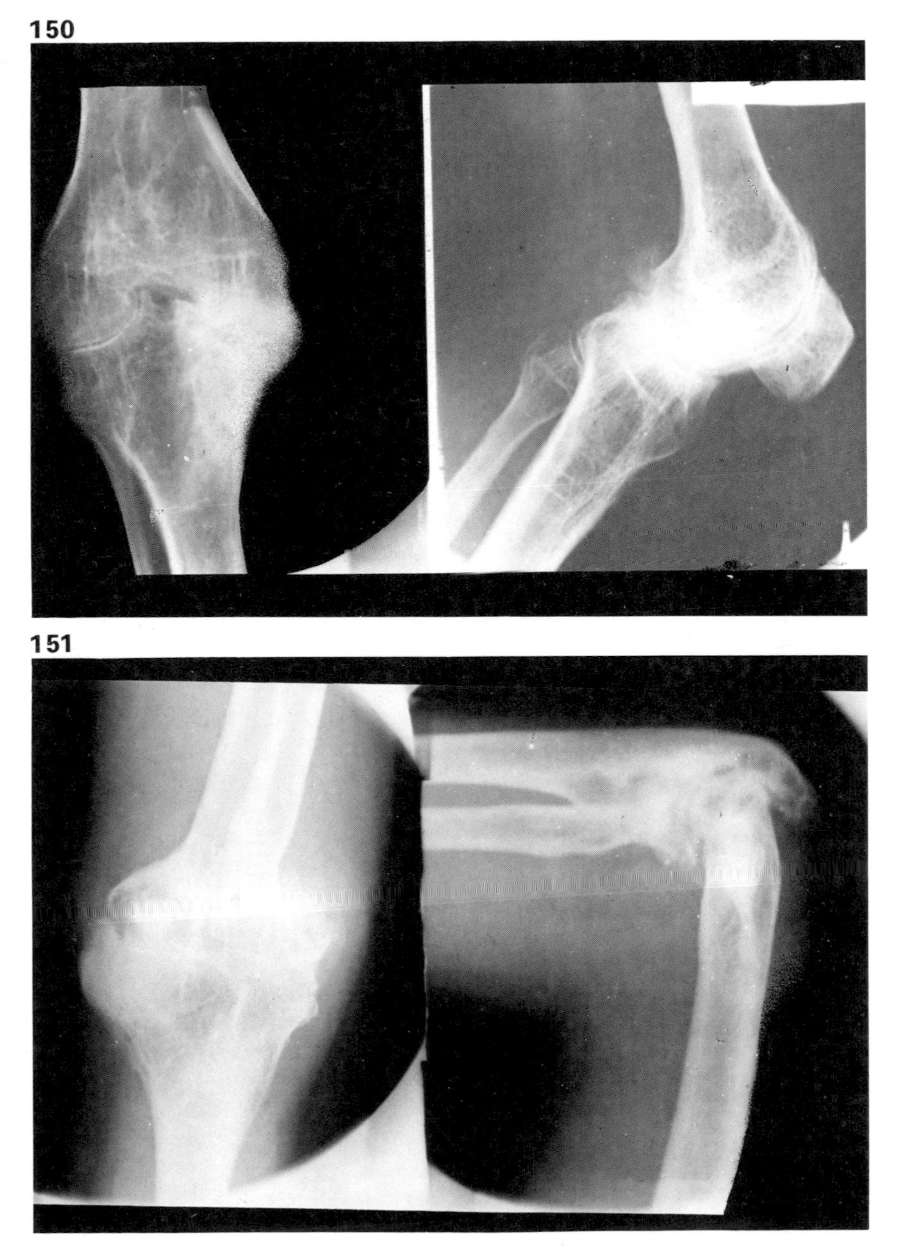

Index

(The references printed in **bold** *type are to picture and caption numbers, those in light type are to page numbers.)*